the **book** of
korean
self-care

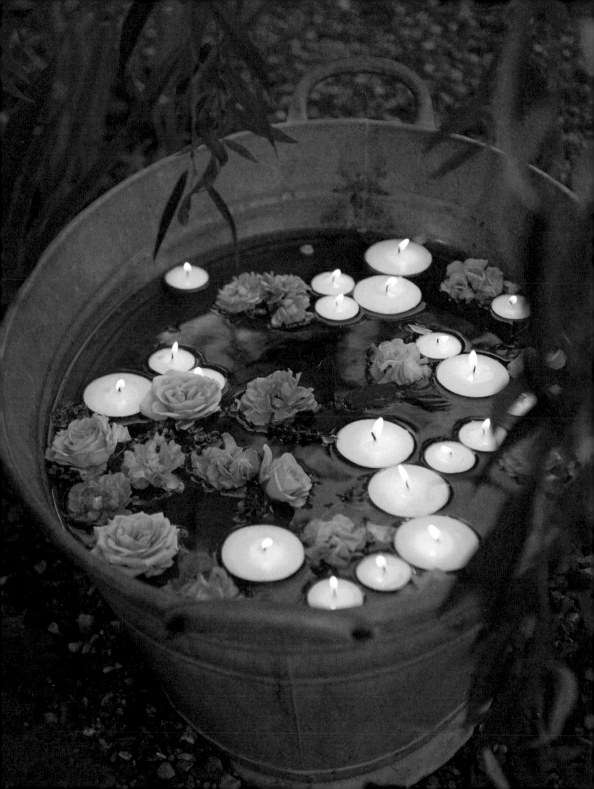

the **book** of
korean
self-care

K-beauty, healing foods, traditional medicine,
mindfulness, and much more

isa kujawski

CICO BOOKS
LONDON NEW YORK

This book is dedicated to:
My grandfather who cherished me,
My aunt who looked after me,
My brother who guided me,
And most of all, my mother who selflessly loves me.

Published in 2023 by CICO Books
An imprint of Ryland Peters & Small Ltd
20–21 Jockey's Fields   341 E 116th St
London   New York
WC1R 4BW   NY 10029

www.rylandpeters.com

10 9 8 7 6 5 4 3 2 1

A CIP catalog record for this book is
available from the Library of Congress
and the British Library.

ISBN: 978-1-80065-204-0

Printed in China

Designer: Geoff Borin
Commissioning editor: Kristine Pidkameny
In-house editor: Jenny Dye
Art director: Sally Powell
Creative director: Leslie Harrington
Production manager: Gordana Simakovic
Publishing manager: Penny Craig

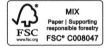

MIX
Paper | Supporting
responsible forestry
FSC® C008047

Notes

• The information in this book is not
intended to replace diagnosis of illness
or ailments, or healing or medicine.
Always consult your doctor or other
health professional in the case of illness
or for dietary advice.

• Both American (Imperial plus US cups)
and British (Metric) are included in these
recipes for your convenience; however,
it is important to work with one set of
measurements only and not alternate
between the two within a recipe.

• All spoon measurements are level unless
otherwise specified. A teaspoon is 5ml,
a tablespoon is 15ml.

• All eggs are large (US) or medium (UK).

contents

introduction

I grew up in a multicultural, overwhelmingly Asian neighborhood known as Flushing within Queens, New York. Chinese, Indian, and Korean cultures were especially well-represented (for the sake of brevity, I will be using "Korean" to mean "South Korean" in this book).

My earliest memories were forged within the melting pot of a unique hub that allowed me to feel immersed in my Korean heritage. In my community, it was commonplace for my peers to speak their mother tongue and eat their ethnic foods. As a child, I didn't realize when I was taking casual field trips to see the Statue of Liberty and Ellis Island, that I was a living, breathing, first-generation embodiment of the American Dream.

Although I am of biracial descent, I grew up exclusively surrounded by my Korean mother's culture, so I always felt more Korean than anything else. Korean was my first language and Korean food was a staple in my household, which meant rice and kimchi were sacrosanct, dessert was fresh-cut fruit, and daily family dinners were honored with our Korean mealtime prayer song (see page 42).

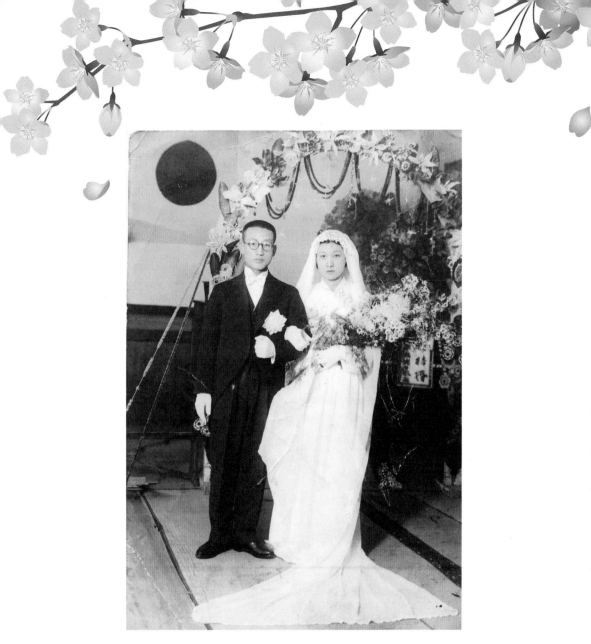

*My grandparents' wedding in Pyongyang, 1941, in what
is now North Korea (this was before Korea split).*

But growing up, for all intents and purposes, "Korean" in America meant much more to our family than our activities of daily living. It represented a collective hero's journey of escaping a war-torn country, settling in South America, and eventually immigrating to the promised land of America to ensure a better life for our family and descendants.

Some of my earliest memories are of attending a Korean church with my Harabuji (grandfather), who was an active member of the Korean community where we lived. Although I lived with Harabuji until I was 18, my relatively limited Korean did not allow us to communicate about his past in depth. I often hear anecdotes from my Umma (mom) about how he grew up in what is now North Korea during the Japanese occupation, which occurred from 1910–1945. After World War II, Korea was split into two zones of occupation—the South under the U.S., and the North under the totalitarian communist leadership of the Soviets. Harabuji was an outspoken activist against communism and consequently targeted. Despite hailing from a wealthy family in Pyongyang, Harabuji and my grandmother left their riches to escape to the South. Umma tells me that at one point, he and my grandmother were separated on their journey out of North Korea and miraculously found each other against all odds.

Eventually, with their nine children in tow, they boarded a boat that led them to Paraguay and ultimately Argentina. After several decades, all but two of my aunts and uncles traveled one by one to the U.S. Umma tells me that she cried all the way to the U.S. as she processed the abandonment of everything familiar to step into the unknown indefinitely.

Umma raised me and my brother while laboring in sweatshops in New York City where she handmade clothing for big-name retailers. Being the breadwinner for her parents as the youngest child meant abandoning her own career dreams. Despite her hard work, she always made a home-cooked meal for our little family and never complained. I love her so much and I am just now beginning to truly appreciate my family's plight and their unending legacy in spite of troubling times.

When I was 18, I joined the United States Navy with the hope of being able to explore my Korean roots further. In 2011, I had the opportunity to be stationed in Seoul, South Korea, where I often worked side by side with the Republic of Korea Navy and was quickly familiarized with my motherland. My friend Paul, a fellow Korean American Naval Officer, would often joke that native Koreans were "KK" (Korean-Korean) and we were "KA" (Korean-American), connoting a comically watered-down version.

And yet, during the two years I lived in Korea, I was able to take a closer look at what it means to be Korean, not only culturally, but mentally. I was privileged to develop friendships with natives who introduced me to the many nuances of the Korean way of life. Furthermore, as a veteran, I learned about the realities of a country torn by conflict and threatened by war—a war that my family fortunately left behind.

Coming full circle, living in Korea meant that I had the opportunity to host my eldest aunt and uncle, both of whom still lived in Argentina at the time and were old enough to have approached adulthood in Korea more than half a century ago. I remember my uncle pointing out the exact building where they grew up, which decades later was surrounded by shops and food stands, within the bustling neighborhood of Namdaemun. Having the opportunity to visit Korea again was something my aunt and uncle only dreamed of, and it was one of my greatest honors to facilitate that opportunity for them.

One thing I was particularly fascinated by was Korea's take on health and wellness. The vast history of Korean food and its healing properties, the popularity of Korean skincare, and the permeating philosophy of natural and health-inspired beauty were themes I wanted to share further with a Western audience. Fast forward ten years, and I have transitioned from active-duty military service, become a functional nutritionist, and opened my own nutrition and wellness practice called Mea Nutrition. Now, having reinvigorated my fascination for Korean health and wellness concepts, I am excited to share them with you.

The tips, modalities, and ideas in this book come from a melding of old and new practices. Heightened worth placed on self-care and mental health among younger generations in Korea have led to the birth of some new mindfulness practices. I am extremely grateful for this, as South Korea has among the highest rates of suicide in the world. I believe normalizing and spreading the value of concepts such as work–life balance and mental decompression, which you'll read about later on, are important steps to lowering the rate of suicide.

The recent popularity of Korean culture worldwide thanks to K-pop and Korean blockbuster hits have led newer Korean words and concepts to be welcomed in to the Western sphere of awareness with open arms. And yet, many ideas presented in this book, such as Korean cuisine and traditional medicine, are steeped in old traditions and permeate the Korean way of life.

As I continue to learn about old and new Korean self-care traditions, I am happy to share with you some of the principles that I have personally grown up with or experienced, and feel have been valuable in my life. It's my hope that you will find some of the tools in this book helpful to your daily life too. I suggest you use this book to introduce yourself to some useful self-care practices and decide which ones suit you. I am a firm believer in bio-individuality—the idea that there is no one-size-fits-all approach—and personal preference when it comes to your health and wellness. So please, make these tools work for you, in whatever way you feel best.

Thank you for your continued interest and willingness to learn with an open mind, and hopefully an open heart.

To the care and keeping of you,

Isa

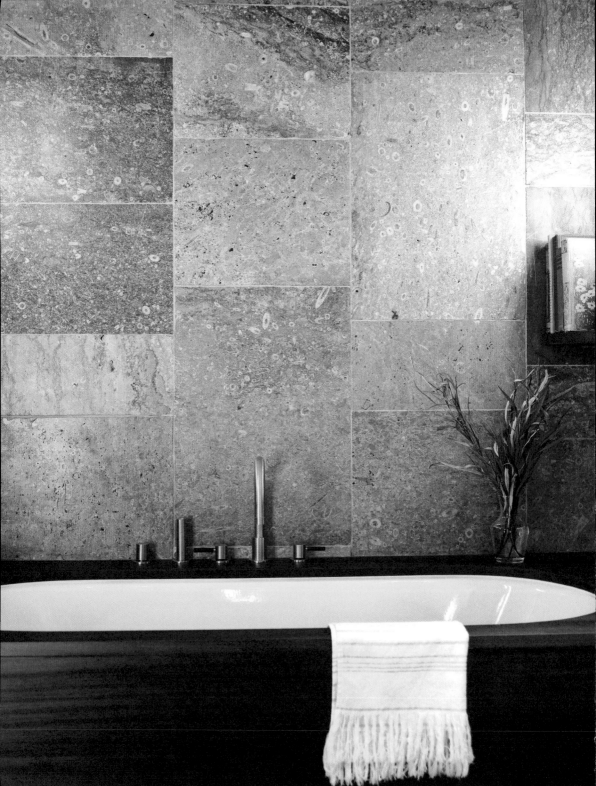

beauty and spa

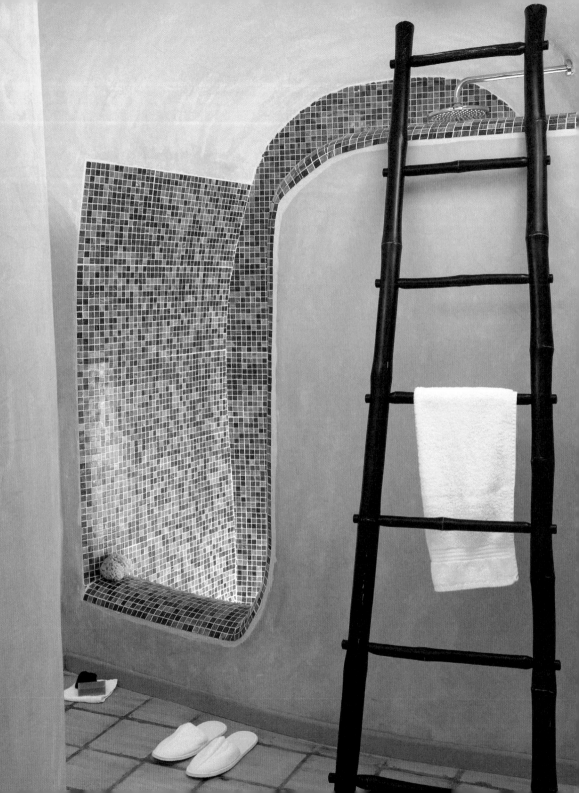

찜질방 jjimjilbang

Imagine a spa mall. A large, earthy, and ambient fortress where you drop your belongings in a locker, change into a soft cotton uniform of a t-shirt and shorts, and decide to sweat, soak, eat, or sleep on heated floors—within walls adorned with crystals, minerals, stones, and wood, with no time limit. You may be excited to learn that these places exist in Korea and in some major cities elsewhere in the world, and they're called jjimjilbangs.

Jjimjilbangs are large Korean bathhouses consisting of kiln saunas called hanjeungmaks (한증막) of various temperatures, hot baths, showers, sleeping rooms, communal areas known as fomentation rooms, and even restaurants. A jjimjilbang may simply sound like a day spa, but to many, they are an escape. They're a place to rest, detoxify, rejuvenate, and just plain chill. They are usually open 24 hours, because rest and relaxation should not be bounded by time.

Other than being havens for decompression, jjimjilbangs are places where the duality of hot and cold can be used for their therapeutic benefits. Steeped in the traditional wisdom of yin and yang (which in Korean, is referred to as um and yang), or the opposing forces of two extremes, thermal (heat/cold) contrast is known to produce sudden changes in the circulatory system to promote healing. This is important to Koreans who emphasize enhanced circulation and blood flow as essential to vitality.

There are several ways in which the amenities of jjimjilbang can be used for hot and cold therapy. However, one does not necessarily need to have access to one of these establishments to experience the therapeutic effects of contrasting temperatures.

therapeutic tubs

Jjimjilbangs are typically furnished with hot and cold therapeutic tubs which patrons may alternate between. This same concept can be practiced by switching between a pool and a jacuzzi a few times. We all know the comfort of stepping into a jacuzzi after the pool gets a little too cold, and vice versa. Alternatively, one may fill a bathtub with ice water and subsequently take a hot bath to experience temperature extremes.

hot and cold saunas

Some jjimjilbangs also house cold saunas that work as a contrast to the very hot temperatures of a hot sauna. This experience can be replicated by stepping in and out of a dry sauna.

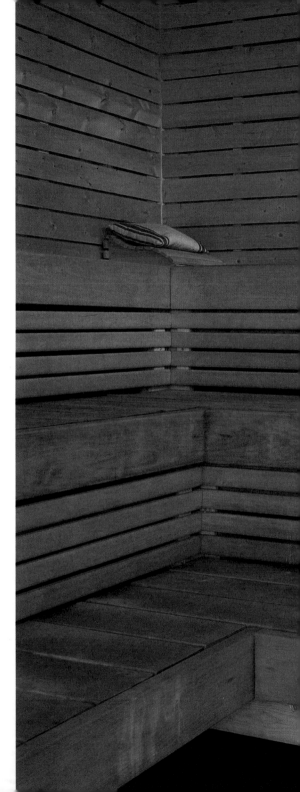

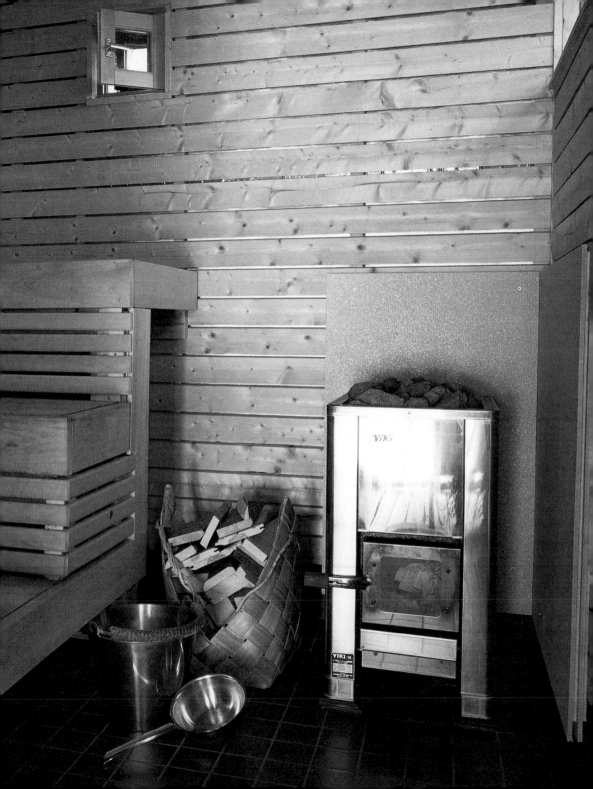

반신욕 ban-shin-yok

Ban-shin-yok, or "half bath," is a Korean bathing technique intended to promote circulation and thus induce a number of healing benefits. This is another ritual that aims to maximize the therapeutic effects of hot and cold. During this process, a hot bath is filled halfway so that the body is exposed to air from the belly button up, while the rest of the body sits in hot water.

The opposing temperatures between the two halves of the body are thought to stimulate blood flow and help alleviate chronic muscle and joint pain, calm the nervous system, and even provide digestive benefits by drawing blood to the core. This elevation of core temperature may also help you break a sweat, aiding in the elimination of toxins and impurities.

This simple bathing ritual can be easily practiced at home, especially after a hard day of work or directly before a night of restful sleep.

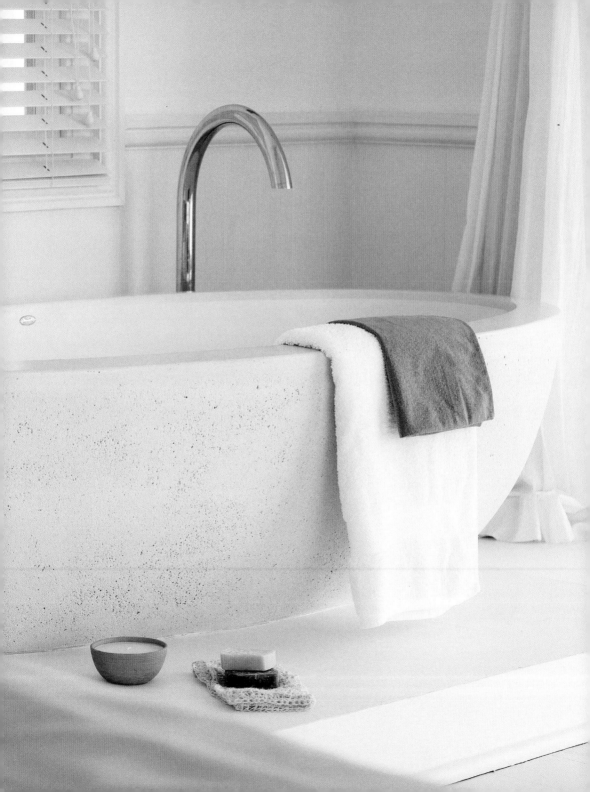

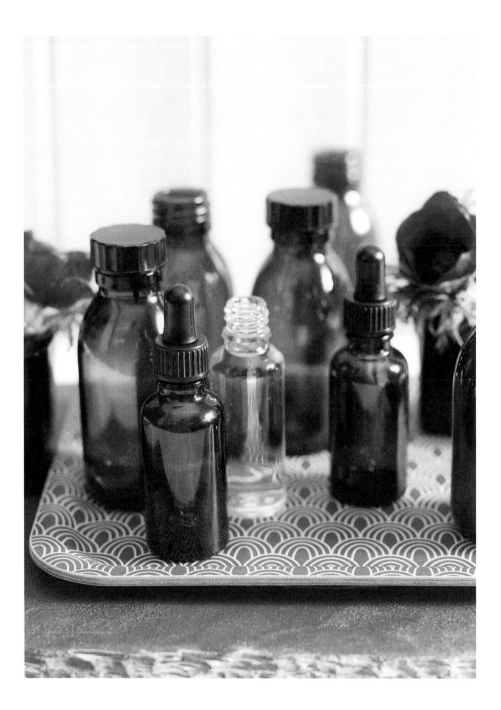

ban-shin-yok in three steps

1 Fill a bath with just enough hot water that the surface hits right below the belly button.

2 Enhance your experience by playing some relaxing music, adding a few drops of essential oils to the bath, or dimming the lights. Remember, self-care should be a harmonious act between mind and body.

3 Remain in the bath for at least 30–45 minutes to reap the benefits of ban-shin-yok. Remember to keep the entire upper body exposed to the air, including the arms.

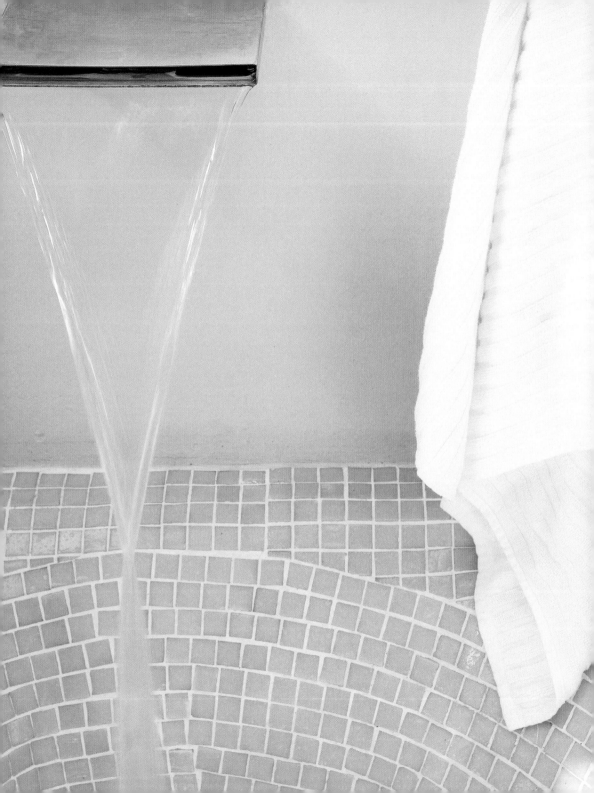

세신 seshin

Seshin is a Korean skin-cleansing ritual that involves scrubbing and exfoliating the body of dead skin to uncover a fresh layer of dermis.

When I was a small child, I remember my mother would have me tightly grasp my opposite forearm in the shower after my skin was moistened and apply friction by rubbing my forearm to and fro. Small gray rolls of dead skin would appear, known as "dde" (때). I would repeat this process on other parts of my body, and this was a regular part of my shower routine.

Although I did this with my bare hands, it is traditionally done with a scrubbing cloth of sandpapery texture after soaking yourself in hot water.

In Korea, seshin is so key that there are ladies known as "ddemiris" (때밀이) or more recently "seshin-sas" (세신사), or scrubbing mistresses, who are employed in jjimjilbangs, or Korean spas (see page 15).

benefits of seshin

o **Circulation and glowing skin:** Seshin reveals soft, supple skin that is better able to absorb nutrients. It also stimulates cell turnover and activates circulation to promote the production of fresh, new skin.

o **Detoxification and drainage:** Seshin clears and opens up pores on the skin's surface, and aids them in releasing waste from the body. It also massages the lymph nodes, stimulating lymphatic drainage, a natural process which transports waste away from the tissues to the lymph nodes to be filtered out.

o **Waste removal:** Sweating is one of the three key modes of detoxification, meaning the skin is constantly accumulating waste that builds up among dead skin. Seshin aids in thoroughly removing this waste.

an at-home seshin routine

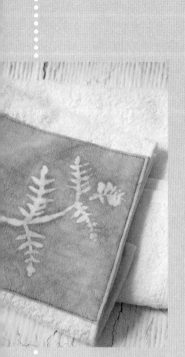

1 Acquire an exfoliating glove or mitt, which you can most likely find in the beauty aisle of most department stores. If you want a genuine Korean exfoliating mitt, a simple internet search will most likely give you options for where to purchase them online. Alternatively, a Korean grocer should also carry them.

2 Sit in a hot bath for at least 30 minutes. Short on time? Practicing seshin at the tail end of a hot shower will do the trick. This will help loosen up dead skin cells.

3 Take your exfoliating mitt or glove and scrub your whole body. Don't forget your belly button, your ankles, and around your ears!

4 Enjoy how refreshingly invigorated your skin feels!

Note: Seshin is best practiced no more than once a week. Over-exfoliating the skin can be damaging and painful, and disturb the skin's delicate microbiome and protective barrier.

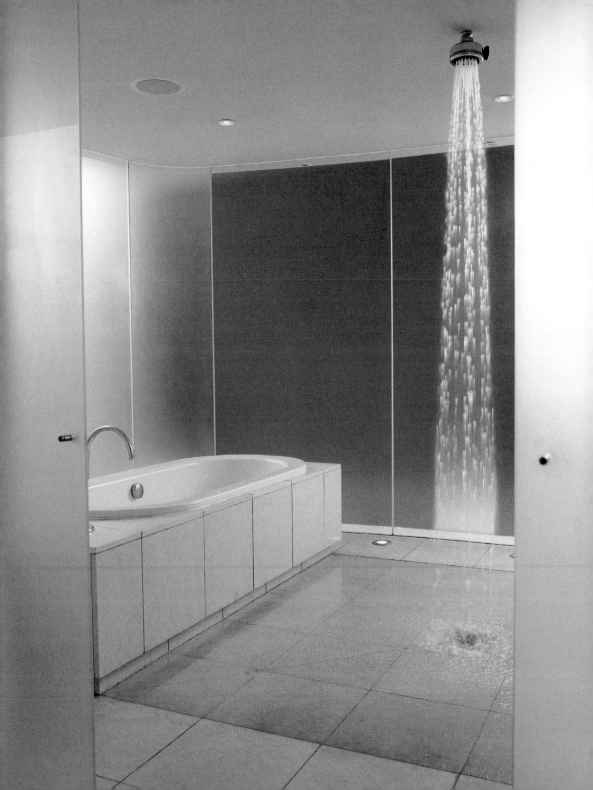

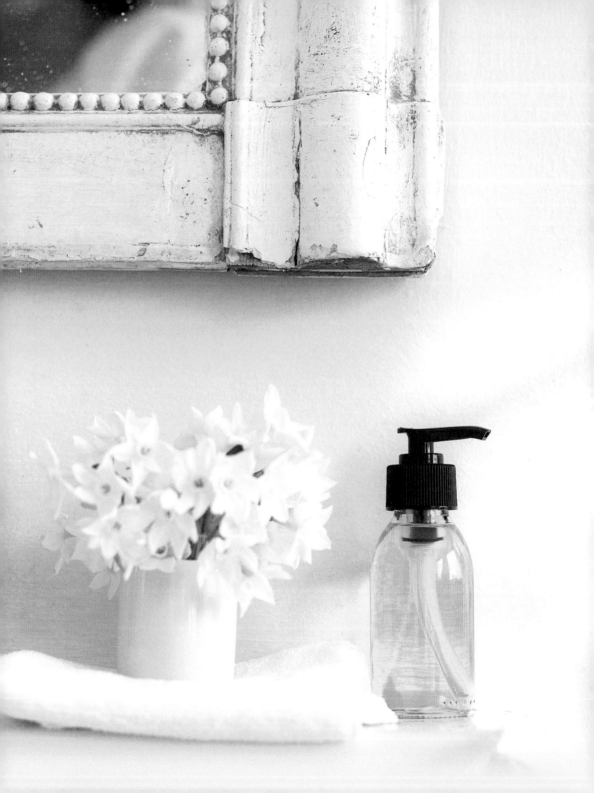

피부 관리 skincare

When thinking of Korean beauty, think skincare and not make up. To Koreans, healthy skin *is* one's natural makeup.

Skincare is a staple practice in K-beauty, emphasizing the health and youthfulness of one's skin above all else. Korean skincare is all about prevention and the maintenance of youth, rather than the more Western ideals of masking or covering up existing damage.

Look at any Korean advertisement, and the model, whether male or female, will have flawless, even-toned skin, seemingly unscathed by the aging effects of the sun. In Korea, skin is thought to be most beautiful when it exudes the quality of luminosity, encompassing moisture, dewiness, and a supreme glowing essence. Koreans aptly use the term "chok chok" (촉촉) to describe this type of skin complexion.

Although some Korean skincare regimens are notorious for having upwards of 10 steps, there are several staple elements that most routines have in common. Of course, these elements may vary based on one's personal skin type. Here are some elements that you can look for when crafting your own skincare regimen.

Cleanser

Korean skincare begins with cleansing, or drawing out impurities from the skin. Typically, an oil-based cleanser is gently massaged into the skin. Oil-based cleansers have the dual benefit of cleansing the skin without stripping it of its natural moisture. They are also very useful because debris and makeup are usually soluble and easily melted away with oil. A recently popularized skincare trend is "double cleansing," which involves cleansing the skin twice by following up an oil-based cleanser with a water-based one to remove any excess dirt and oil residue. Cleansing in two steps is generally considered more thorough in prepping the skin to receive and absorb follow-on products.

Common ingredients: coconut oil, jojoba oil, castor oil

Exfoliator

Sloughing away dead skin that builds up on the skin's surface is an integral part of keeping the skin fresh and renewed. This step is also important as it cleans out debris from pores, especially in the t-zone of the nose and surrounding areas. When pores fill up with oil, also known as sebum, they can become clogged and enlarged over time. Although exfoliation is a key component of Korean skincare, it is typically conducted only one to two times a week, or as needed. More than that is too abrasive for the skin. Exfoliating agents usually include acids, which work by promoting skin-cell turnover.

Common ingredients: salicylic acid, glycolic acid

Toner

Toners offer a last-ditch way to remove remaining residue on the skin while balancing its pH and restoring moisture.

Common ingredients: hyaloronic acid, mineral water, rose water

Essence

Essences are water-based products that normally have a refreshing fragrance and are concentrated with beneficial active ingredients to rehydrate the skin while enhancing the complexion. With their relatively thin and lightweight quality, essences are meant to easily penetrate the skin. The ingredients vary from brand to brand, making essences quite ambiguous and up to the discretion of the user. Although some people may find this step essential, others consider it redundant.

Common ingredients: glycerin, glycol, botanical plant extracts

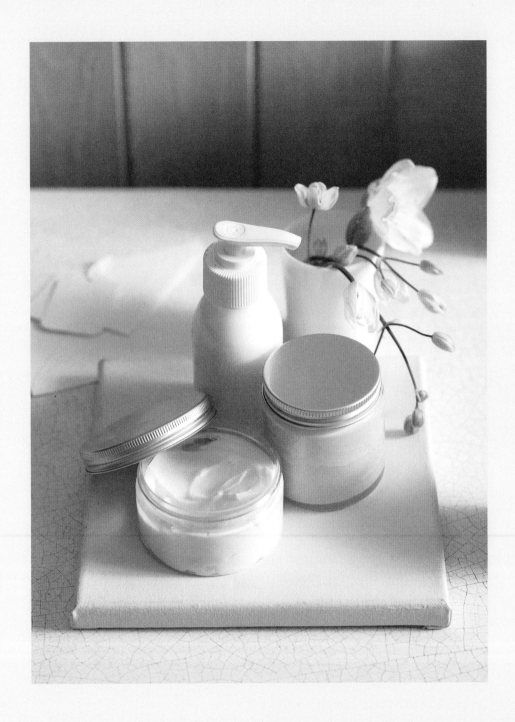

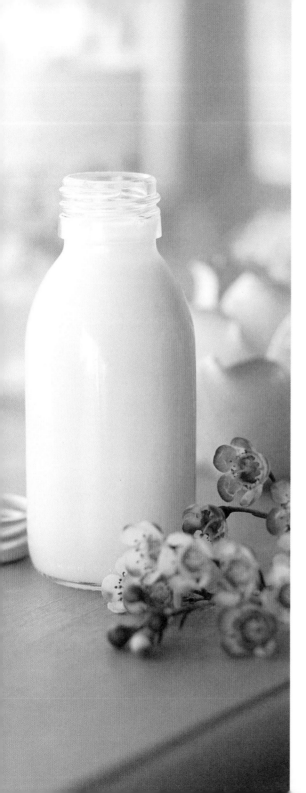

Serums and treatments

At this point, the skin should be well cleansed and prepared to receive serums that target individualized needs and goals including acne, fine lines, hyperpigmentation, and wrinkles.

Common ingredients: retinol/retinoids, vitamin C, niacinamide, tea tree oil, hyaluronic acid

Eye creams

Because of the delicate nature of the skin around the eye area, special products are made just for the eyes. These products are usually designed to address fine lines, puffiness, and dark circles.

Common ingredients: Coenzyme Q-10, vitamins C, E, K, hyaluronic acid

Sheet masks

Sheet masks are quite prevalent in Korea and are considered both a skincare practice as well as a relaxing ritual. A sheet mask is basically a wet clothlike sheet with cutouts for your eyes that has been treated with product, much like an essence. The idea is to relax with a sheet mask resting on your face for about 15–30 minutes to allow the skin to absorb nutrients from the sheet mask. Lying down or reclining on your back to allow the mask to rest on the face gives you no choice but to relax and unwind while the sheet's active ingredients work their magic.

Common ingredients: green tea extract, plant botanicals

Moisturizer

No skincare regimen is complete without a soothing moisturizer to seal in hydration and promote a plump and dewy complexion. Moisturizers will often be for either night or day—evening moisturizers are usually thicker, richer, and promote overnight repair, while day moisturizers are lighter and often contain SPF. Individuals are often advised to gently pat moisturizers on their face and neck to avoid rubbing and consequently tugging and stretching one's delicate skin.

Common ingredients: ginseng, vitamin E, propolis

Sun protection

To the prevention-conscious K-beauty connoisseur, sun protection is a must. The sun is considered to be the number one culprit of premature aging. This step usually comes directly before or after applying a daily moisturizer. Sun-protection products contain either mineral protectants such as titanium dioxide and zinc oxide, which rest on the skin's surface to act as a physical shield, or chemical protectants like avobenzone and octinoxate, which are absorbed into the skin. In the last decade, products known as BB creams and CC creams have become more prevalent. These products combine the function of multiple skincare products into one, including moisturizing, antiaging, and evening skin tone, while also containing SPF.

Common ingredients: zinc oxide, titanium dioxide

"Skip care" approach

Luckily, the tide is shifting towards minimalism when it comes to Korean skincare. Although you'll hear legends of ten-step skincare regimens, that's not always realistic and accessible, and it doesn't necessarily mean that all ten steps are administered every single day in sequential order. The term "skip care" caters to the vast majority of people who want something effective yet simple. Minimal skincare entails using products that consolidate ingredients without compromising their effectiveness. For example, you could use a day moisturizer that includes SPF, or a serum that doubles as an essence, or a foundation that includes moisturizer and antiaging ingredients.

K-beauty-inspired DIY face masks

When I lived in Korea, I received a few facials that made me realize how relaxing and invigorating face masks can feel. Here are some K-beauty-inspired face masks that you can make at home with a few simple ingredients. Make these masks by mixing the ingredients in a small bowl, applying to cleansed skin, and leaving on for 15–30 minutes. Rinse with warm water and pat your skin dry.

Nourishing green tea mask

¼ mashed avocado (hydrating and moisturizing)

1 tsp freshly squeezed lemon juice (evens out skin tone, cleanses, and reduces appearance of dark spots and scars)

1 tsp matcha powder (antioxidizing)

Soothing honey and aloe vera mask

1 tsp coconut oil (cleansing and nourishing)

2 tbsp aloe vera (soothing)

1 tbsp honey (moisturizing and cleanses pores)

Detoxifying clay mask

2 tbsp bentonite clay (antibacterial and anti-inflammatory)

2 tbsp apple cider vinegar (cider vinegar) (antimicrobial and antifungal)

1 drop tea tree essential oil (optional)

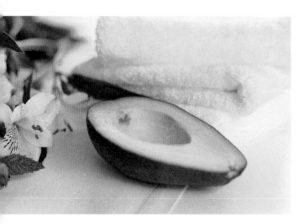

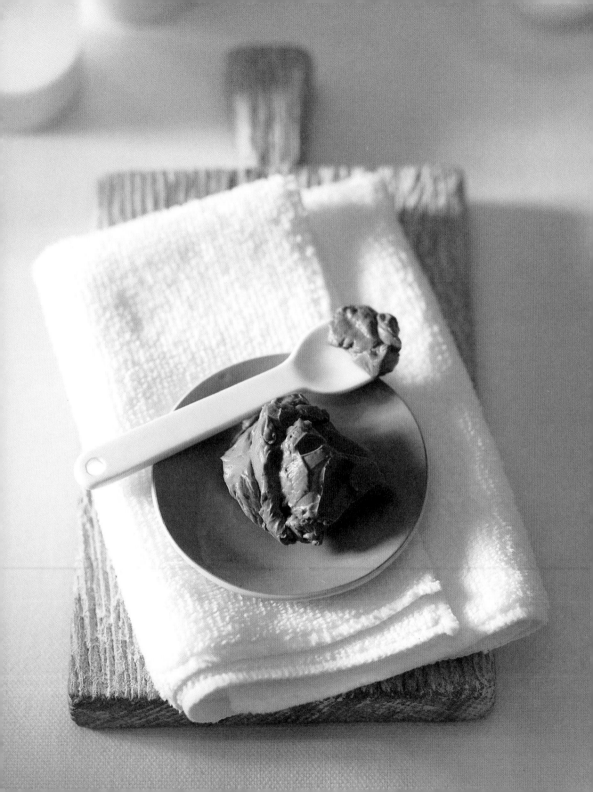

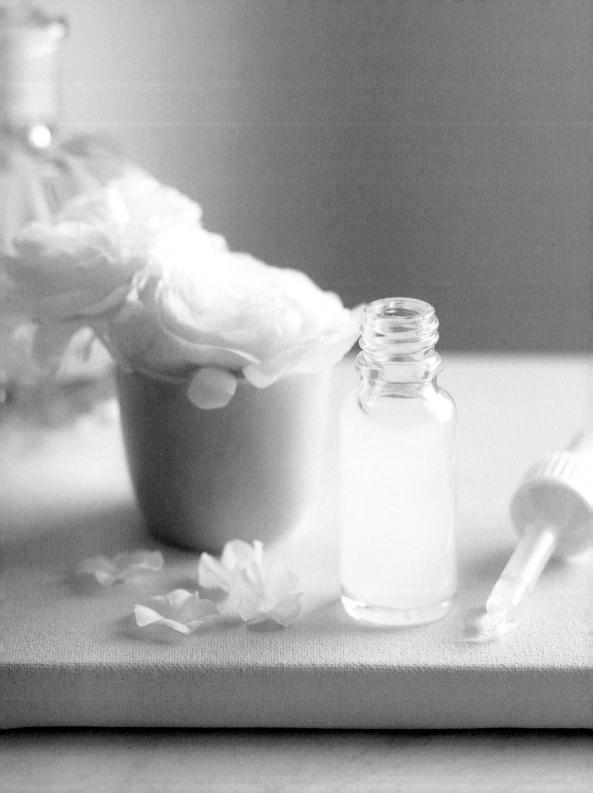

creating your own skincare routine

1 Don't stress

There's no doubt that creating a skincare routine can get overwhelming with so many different products available. When you start out, focus on the key basics: a cleanser, serum, moisturizer, and sunscreen. When drying, pat, don't rub.

2 Keep an open mind

I suggest consulting with a few aestheticians to get their take on your skin type and the best products for your goals and budget. They can guide you towards options, resources, and provide general education so you're better equipped to navigate your choices. Many skincare shops hire aestheticians as store associates, so if you're browsing and someone asks "may I help you?," ask questions!

3 Honor your unique skin

Your skin is unique to you. Just because something works wonders for your friend, it doesn't mean it will for you too.

4 Be smart

Skincare products can get expensive, so gather samples to test or ask about a store's return policy. You want to have the option to return lightly used products if they don't agree with your skin.

5 Just start

You don't have to wait until you find a forever product to start your skincare routine. There's no harm in choosing well-reviewed products, using them consistently, and trying another one! It took me many years to finally find products I know, love, and trust but it was well worth the search.

화장 makeup

If there's one word that sums up the ideal makeup "look" in Korea, it's youthful. While the Western world may prioritize covering up and contouring, K-beauty emphasizes a "no makeup" look with a dewy, radiant, "glassy" finish. For a less-is-more look, try these techniques.

Consider a lip stain
Ditch the lipliner and bold lip colors. Lip stains are all about enhancing your natural color without a thick layer of product.

Go for a dewy rather than matte finish
It's all about looking fresh, radiant, and hydrated, kind of like a dolphin. Try BB or CC creams that double as skincare.

Soften the arch on your brows
Young, innocent, and soft is the name of the game.

Tightline your eyes
Instead of drawing a bold line with eyeliner, line the inner lash line itself to enhance the eyes, not change them.

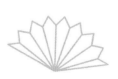

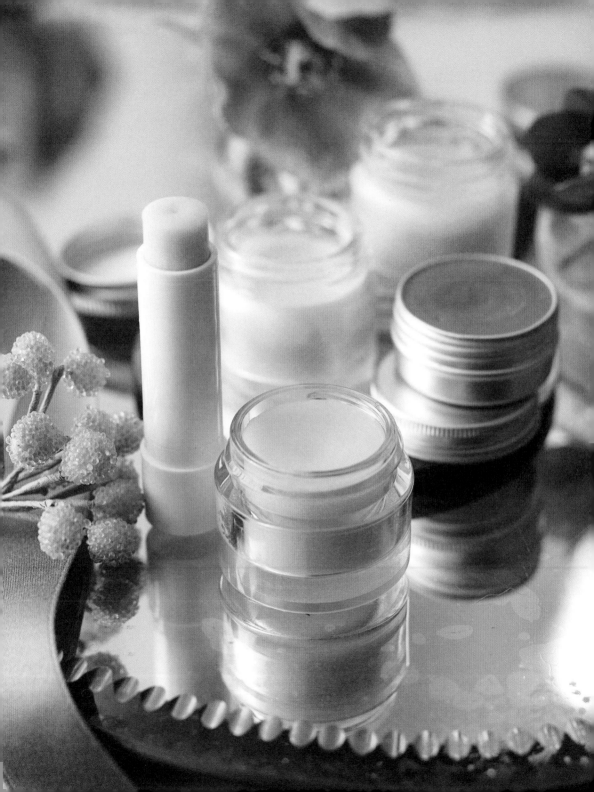

이너 뷰티

inner beauty

Koreans realize that outer beauty is more than just skincare and makeup—it's a reflection of inner health. Due to this, the term "inner beauty" has been coined recently as its own K-beauty category, and emphasizes functional foods and supplements to address problems such as acne, fine lines, and skin irritation. Active ingredients may include collagen and probiotics.

Inner beauty has become so popular that most Koreans consume some sort of functional health product such as gummies and drink mixes. This does not mean you have to go out and buy a bunch of products that tout health claims. In fact, as a nutritionist, I would advise against it! Here are some nutrition essentials that may help your body radiate outer beauty.

Water

Drink plenty of water to keep hydrated. Water helps your body flush out toxins, and helps your skin maintain its moisture and elasticity. No amount of product will help your skin look as good as water can!

Functional foods

Regularly eating nutrient-dense whole foods will help your body maintain a diverse nutritional profile and provide antioxidant benefits. Nutrient-dense whole foods include fruits and vegetables, protein, and healthy fats.

Multivitamin

Consider a multivitamin to fill in any nutritional gaps that you may not be getting from food. Different vitamins and minerals play key roles in virtually every process in your body—this includes processes that keep your skin looking its best.

Consult a dietitian or nutritionist

The upfront cost of consulting with a dietitian or a nutritionist you trust to help you choose more specialized supplements may make up for wasted money buying needless or even harmful products.

In the next few chapters, you'll learn more about healing, nutritious Korean foods. The idea of foods playing a functional role is central to the Korean way of life. So if the idea of inner beauty resonates with you, read on.

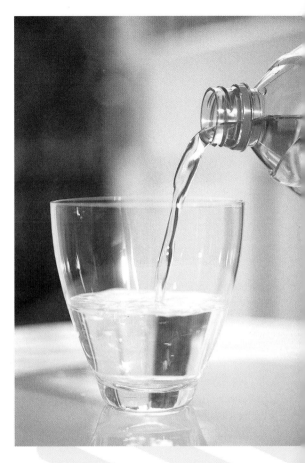

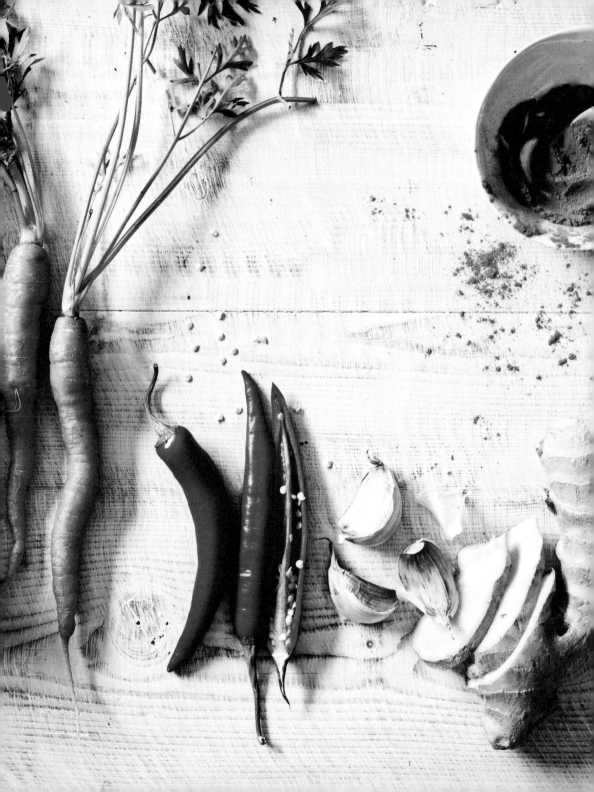

healing foods

Growing up in a Korean household meant that all dinner meals were consumed together as a family with little exception. For me, this consisted of my mother, brother, aunt, and grandfather. We all sat at the dining table and started each meal by singing a mealtime prayer song. Then, we would wait for my grandfather, the eldest, to take his first bite before starting to eat ourselves. Although the song is intended for children, we never stopped singing it until I was 18 and left home. To this day, I sometimes sing it in my head as a way to practice gratitude for my food.

mealtime prayer song

Lyrics in Korean:

날마다 우리에게 양식을 주시는
은혜로우신 하나님 참 감사합니다.
아~멘

Phonetic pronunciation:

nahl-mah-dah oo-ree eh-geh yang-shik-eul joo-shi-neun eun-heh-ro oo-shin hah-nah-neem jeul gam-sah-hahb-nee-dah

ah-men

Translation in English:

For the meal that you provide for us daily
We joyfully thank our Gracious God.
A-men

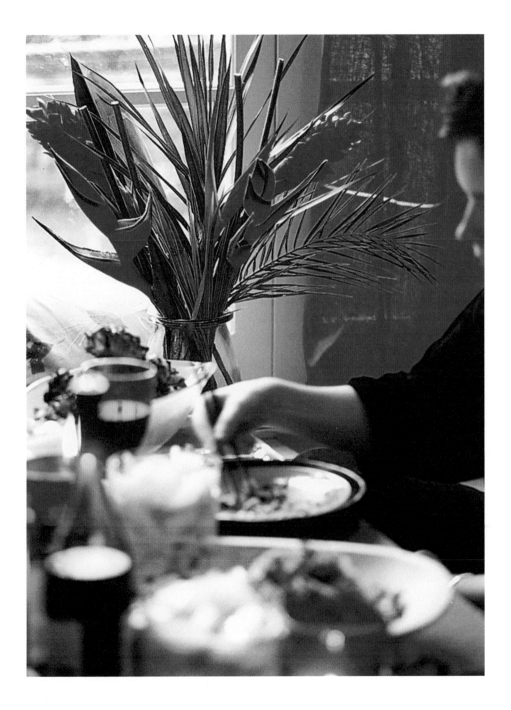

한식 hansik

Hansik refers to the format of traditional Korean cuisine. By design, hansik includes several dishes that cover the bases of a healthful meal.

Hansik is my absolute favorite style of eating because it's so satisfying. When I stop and think about why, the word that occurs to me is balance. Hansik includes just the right balance of hot and cold, savory and sweet, soft and crunchy. It is nourishing enough to feel satisfying yet light enough to keep you energetic.

Of course, the topic of hansik and its accompanying recipes could fill up several books on their own, but here are the basic elements of hansik.

반찬 Banchan

Banchan are small side dishes that accompany a traditional home-cooked meal. These usually include kimchi and marinated vegetables, or more dense items such as eggs, fish, and potatoes. Ruth Tobias, author of a Thrillist article about banchan sums it up perfectly:

"They represent a category unto themselves: snacks-within-a-meal that function as complements, contrasts, and condiments all at once."

국 Guk

Guk translates as soup. Soups add a brothy, savory, and warm comfort to the meal, complementing the rice perfectly. Guk may have a lighter, mild flavor or a deeper, spicy taste depending on the variety.

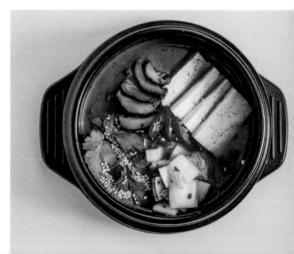

밥 Bap

Bap is rice—an essential element in a hansik meal. Rice acts as the base of a meal, soaking up the saltiness of banchan and guk, creating a harmonious balance in the meal. Korean rice is usually short grain, and more classical versions may also include several grains and legumes mixed together such as black sweet rice, barley, peas, and red beans.

You don't have to know much about Korean food just yet to create a hansik-inspired meal format. Just focus on balance. Create a tray of your own that includes a small bowl of rice, a little bowl of broth, and several crunchy vegetables or salads, with a side of protein such as fish, tofu, or beans. You'll find that creating a variety of flavors and textures within a meal creates ritual and satisfaction.

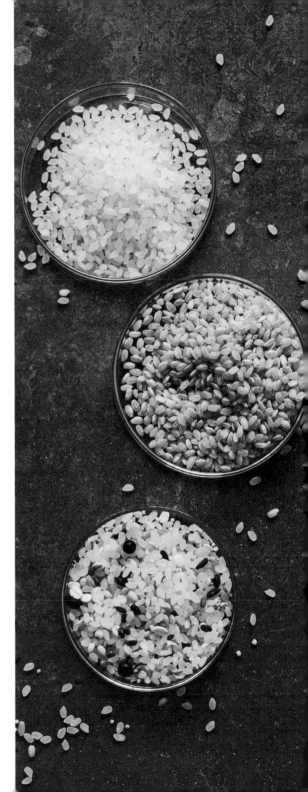

김치 | kimchi

Kimchi is not simply a popular food item in Korea, it is a necessity. Go to any household and you will find kimchi served alongside every dish like a comforting sidekick. To most Koreans, a meal is seldom complete without the all-too-familiar pungent, salty, and tangy notes that kimchi provides. The presence of kimchi is healing unto itself.

Although one may think of a singular dish when hearing "kimchi," it really refers to fermented vegetables, encompassing several hundred types, combined with different ingredients, varying by region, season, and household. Many Koreans find comfort in their mothers' original recipes, passed down through generations.

Kimchi's influence has permeated cultures, coasts, and continents. If you ask any foreigner to think of Korean food, they will usually think of kimchi. Today, kimchi is found in many Western grocery stores, and spotlighted as a featured ingredient in fusion dishes from fries to tacos.

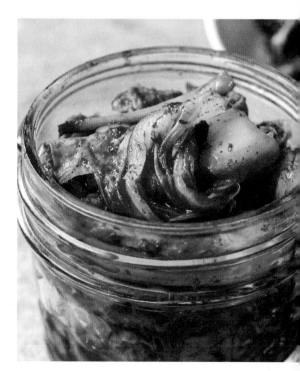

the health benefits of kimchi

As a functional nutritionist myself, I am constantly educating my clients on the benefits of fermented foods. Kimchi is teeming with beneficial bacteria known as probiotics, which are a byproduct of the fermentation process involving lactic acid bacteria. Fermented kimchi contains hundreds of strains of probiotics. The benefits of probiotics are plentiful, including alleviation of digestive issues, restoration of proper gut bacteria balance, and support of mental and immune health. Depending on the variety, kimchi is also rich in nutrients including vitamins A, C, K, folate, potassium, and calcium.

the four steps of kimchi-making

Homemade fermented kimchi-making is a labor of love, involving several steps that can span from days to months.

Salt brining
This step involves cutting the vegetables and coating them in salt, which opens up their pores and draws out excess water. Salt also creates an unfavorable environment for unfriendly microorganisms. The vegetables become pleasantly tender and ready to receive their delicious flavors.

Seasoning
Generally, kimchi's distinct flavor is a product of both fermentation and several key spices including garlic, ginger, and gochugaru (고춧가루), or chili pepper powder. Sugar may also be added to the mix to promote both flavor and fermentation.

Fermenting
The seasoned vegetables are then densely packed into jars and stored in a cool dark place, allowing them to begin the fermentation process, where bacteria metabolize the carbohydrates in the vegetables into lactic acid. The kimchi becomes nice and bubbly in this phase, since carbon dioxide is a byproduct of fermentation!

Storing
Historically, kimchi was stored in giant stone pots called onngis (옹기) that were buried underground. Today, kimchi is usually refrigerated in glass containers. Some modern Korean households even have "kimchi refrigerators" that keep kimchi at optimal temperatures through the different stages of its aging process.

kimchi through the seasons

Autumn/winter kimchi

Autumn and winter kimchis are typically fermented and exhibit a rich depth of flavor. Kimjang (김장) refers to the autumn season of making and sharing kimchi in preparation for the winter months. During the warmer months, essential ingredients such as seafood, salt, and red chili peppers are procured in preparation. Kimjang is not just about kimchi-making, it's about solidarity.

막김치 mak kimchi recipe

(Easy kimchi—see the picture on page 46)

Mak kimchi is made with napa cabbage. It's a simplified take on more complicated classic kimchi recipes—hence the name "mak," which means roughly or carelessly.

1–2 heads napa cabbage, or 4lb/1.8kg in total

2 tbsp kosher salt

2 cloves garlic, minced

1-in (2.5-cm) piece fresh ginger, peeled and finely grated

2 tbsp fish sauce (optional or replace with soy sauce for vegans)

¼ cup/2oz/55g gochugaru (Korean red chili flakes)

1½ tsp sugar (optional)

3 scallions (spring onions), roughly chopped

Makes approx. 4lb/1.8kg kimchi

1 Wash, dry, and roughly cut the napa cabbage into 2-in (5-cm) pieces.

2 In a large bowl, evenly coat the cabbage with the salt and let it sit for 50–60 minutes.

3 By now, the cabbage should be tender and bendable. Rinse the cabbage with water and drain the excess water.

4 Mix all the remaining ingredients except the scallions (spring onions) in a bowl to form the paste. Add small amounts of water as needed to form a smooth yet thick paste.

5 Mix the cabbage with the seasoning paste and scallions in a large bowl until the cabbage is evenly coated.

6 Tightly pack the kimchi in a clean medium-sized jar or airtight container and add ¼ cup/2fl oz/55ml water on top to fill it to the top and make it airtight. It is not necessary to sterilize the jar or container as the process of lacto fermentation will control the microbial environment.

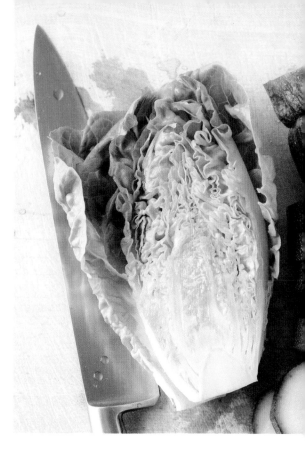

7 Place the jar or container on a plate and let it sit for one to three days at room temperature before putting it in the fridge. Once refrigerated, it is ready to eat. It should last in the fridge for 3–6 months. Enjoy!

Spring/summer kimchi

Like spring kimchis, many summer kimchis are made instantly without the need for fermentation, using in-season vegetables such as cucumbers and radishes.

오이 무침 oi muchim recipe

(Instant cucumber kimchi)

This easy, instant cucumber kimchi is light and crunchy, and may be served as a great addition to any meal.

2 English cucumbers

sea salt, to taste

2 garlic cloves, minced

1 tbsp sesame oil

3 tbsp gochugaru (Korean red pepper flakes)*

1 tsp sesame seeds

½ tsp sugar*

2 tbsp rice vinegar

optional vegetable garnishes (2oz/55g each): julienned carrots, sliced scallions (spring onions), Asian chives

*Amount of sugar and spices may be adjusted to suit your taste

Makes enough kimchi to fill a small to medium food container

1 Thinly slice cucumbers into slices around 1⁄16–1⁄8in (2–3mm) thick.

2 Sprinkle the cucumbers with the salt and set aside for 10–15 minutes.

3 Rinse the cucumbers with cold water, then strain and gently squeeze out excess water using your hands. Do not over-squeeze and take care not to break the cucumber pieces.

4 In a large bowl, mix together the remaining ingredients including the optional vegetable garnishes. Mix in the cucumber slices before serving.

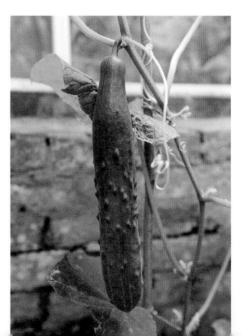

미역국 miyeok guk

(korean seaweed soup)

One of my favorite soups growing up was miyeok guk, which translates as seaweed soup. This savory, briny soup has a distinctive and delicious flavor, owing to the edible seaweed that is central to the dish. Although many people who have not tried this may be put off by the idea of seaweed soup, I personally think most would be pleasantly surprised by its rich umami, or savory, flavor profile.

Although miyeok guk is regularly consumed by Korean households, it is also adoringly known as birthday soup because it is customarily served to mothers who have just given birth. Some even consume it as many as three times daily for a month after giving birth. Koreans embrace the tradition of serving miyeok guk on birthdays to pay homage to their mothers.

The nutrients provided by the seaweed contain myriad "superfood" health benefits that are believed to help new mothers recover and produce abundant breast milk. Miyeok is packed with vitamins and minerals including iodine, calcium, omega 3 fatty acids, B vitamins, potassium, iron, magnesium, vitamins A and C, and fiber. Miyeok is also beneficial to cardiovascular health and immunity.

Note

Although this soup is consumed frequently by new mothers in Korea, new research is finding that seaweed should not be overconsumed because of the copious amounts of iodine it contains, potentially hundreds of times higher than the daily recommended intake depending on the dose. Although iodine is known to be beneficial for thyroid function, too much can have reverse effects for both the mother and baby.

miyeok guk recipe

The best part about this soup is that it is very easy to make and hard to mess up. You can vary the choice of protein to make it to your liking.

1oz/30g dried miyeok (You can find this at Korean groceries—it is typically sold in long bags and appears long and stringy with a deep green hue that looks almost black. Alternatively, you may run a search for miyeok or "dried korean seaweed" and order it online.)

12oz/340g thinly sliced beef brisket (alternatively, you may use a similar amount of seafood, tofu, or chicken)

3 garlic cloves, minced

1½ tbsp soy sauce or tamari

1 tbsp sesame oil

sea salt, to taste

optional added vegetables: ½ onion, sliced; 2 scallions (spring onions), chopped; 1-in (2.5-cm) piece of fresh ginger, peeled and chopped

Serves 4–6

1 Soak the dried miyeok in lukewarm water for 30–60 minutes. The miyeok will multiply in size, so use a medium sized bowl and immerse the seaweed by at least 3in (7.5cm).

2 Rinse the miyeok and use your hands to squeeze out the excess water. Cut into bite-sized pieces.

3 Place the miyeok in a large pot or dutch oven with 6–8 cups/1.4–1.9 liters of water and bring to a boil for 15 minutes with the lid on.

4 Add in the thinly sliced beef brisket or your choice of protein, and continue to boil covered for around 45 minutes. If you are using seafood, add after this time.

5 Stir in remaining ingredients and optional vegetables. Allow to simmer for another 15 minutes before serving.

삼계탕 **samgyetang**

(ginseng chicken soup)

Ginseng chicken soup is my favorite Korean comfort dish. One of my fondest memories of living in Korea is eating this delicious soup in an unsuspecting hole-in-the-wall eatery nestled in an alleyway in the southern port city of Busan. The place was so hidden that you only knew about it by word of mouth. It felt like a speakeasy for the best samgyetang you could eat in your life.

If it were up to me, I would enjoy this dish on the coldest winter day, but Koreans have a unique tradition of consuming this soup on the hottest three days of summer, referred to as sambok (삼복), usually occurring in Korea between mid-July and mid-August. If you don't live in Korea, a fun thing to do may be to look up the climate predictions for the hottest days in your local area. This idea of overcoming heat with more heat in an effort to stay cool is concisely summarized by the saying yi-yeol-chi-yeol (이열치열), which means "fight fire with fire."

Samgyetang contains various ingredients which make this soup a complete, nourishing meal.

Medicinal ingredients

Samgyetang includes ginseng, which contains bioactive ingredients known for their antioxidant and anti-inflammatory properties. Ginseng is among the five most used medicinal herbs in Korea, known to help strengthen the immune system, lower blood sugar, reduce stress, and help fight chronic fatigue. Other beneficial ingredients are ginger, garlic and jujubes. Jujubes are a dried, reddish, and shriveled fruit resembling a date with a mildly sweet and tart flavor and a crispy texture when raw.

Chicken

Samgyetang's main feature is an entire small chicken stuffed with rice. According to the book *Dongui Bogam* compiled by royal physician Heo Jun in the 1600s, chicken increases the body's temperature and digestive power, and ignites energy.

Glutinous rice

According to an article by the Korea Food Research Institute, glutinous rice contains a high proportion of amylopectin, making it easier to digest and absorb with little irritation to the gut wall. It is also rich in vitamins B1, B2, D, and E.

samgyetang recipe

This recipe was adapted from one by the popular Korean food blogger and YouTuber Maangchi.

2 cornish hens or poissons, each weighing less than 2lbs/900g

12 garlic cloves

¾ cup/175g sweet glutinous rice, soaked in water for 1 hour

2 fresh ginseng roots

4 dried jujubes

4 thin slices of peeled fresh ginger

1 onion, sliced

10 cups/80fl oz/2.35 liters store-bought or homemade chicken broth or water

3 scallions (spring onions), chopped sea salt and freshly ground black pepper, to taste.

Serves 2

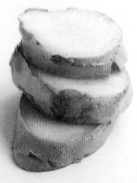

1 Prepare the hens or poissons by rinsing them in cold water. Remove the giblets and trim away excess fat.

2 Stuff the cavity of each hen or poisson with 6 garlic cloves and some of the rice. Leave a little room in the cavity for the rice to expand as it cooks. Tuck the legs into either side of the cavity to secure the contents inside.

3 Place the hens or poissons, along with the ginseng roots, jujubes, ginger, onions, and remaining rice in a large pot with a matching lid, with the chicken broth or water.

4 Cover and boil the contents for 20 minutes on high heat, then lower the heat and cook for another 30 minutes at a low simmer. Remove from the heat and leave to rest for 10–15 minutes before serving.

5 Place each hen into its own bowl along with some of the broth. Evenly distribute the other ingredients between the bowls. Top each bowl with chopped scallions (spring onions) and season with salt and pepper to taste. Serve and enjoy.

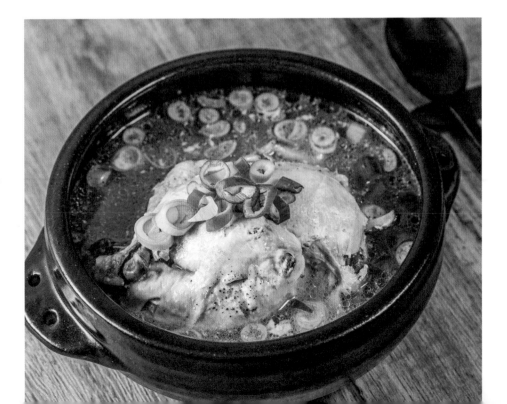

나물 **namul**

(seasoned edible grasses and vegetables)

Namul refers to a variety of edible grasses or plants that are marinated and customarily eaten as banchan (see page 44). The saltiness of the namul is well balanced against rice. If you've ever been to a Korean restaurant before, you're sure to have tried some variety of namul. Some Koreans even know how to forage for these plants in the wild, but it is best to stick to a grocery store or grow them yourself just to be safe (see page 135)!

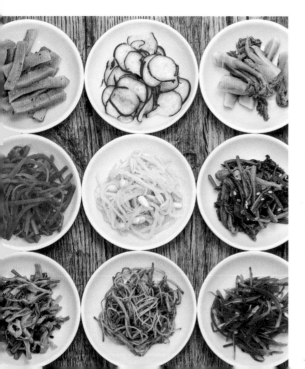

Namul is an essential part of a medicinal Korean meal, as it is rich in fiber and myriad phytochemicals, which are special nutrients found in plant foods. Phytonutrients present a variety of health benefits such as detoxification, lowering inflammation, and enhancing immunity.

The possibilities for namul are endless, as there are so many grasses and vegetables and various parts of them can be used, along with styles of preparation and spices. Below are some of my favorite types of namul.

깻잎 Kkaenip (perilla leaves)

Perilla leaves contain calcium, magnesium, phosphorus, vitamin C, iron, and essential fatty acids. They have been associated with anti-nausea, antiallergic, and anticancer effects.

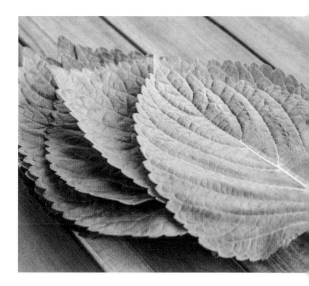

For the seasoning sauce:

½ cup/4fl oz/120ml soy sauce

3 garlic cloves, minced

½ tbsp gochugaru
(Korean chili pepper flakes)

2 scallions (spring onions),
finely chopped

1–2 tsp sugar

approx. 30 perilla leaves, rinsed

short-grain rice—amount required to serve your gathering (any extra perilla leaves can be stored in an airtight container in the refrigerator)

Serve as a banchan
(side dish—see page 44)

1 In a bowl, mix together the ingredients for the seasoning sauce.

2 In a container, stack all of the perilla leaves on top of each other, using a spoon to roughly spread a little bit of sauce on every second leaf. Pour any remaining sauce on top of and around the leaves. Place the lid on the container, refrigerate, and allow at least 48 hours for the leaves to fully absorb the flavor before consuming.

3 To serve, cook the rice according to the packet instructions. Enjoy the perilla leaves by placing a small amount of rice on each leaf, and wrapping the leaf around the rice.

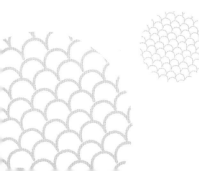

namul (seasoned edible grasses and vegetables) **57**

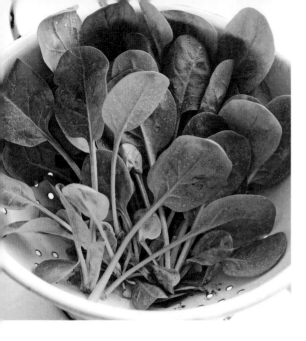

1 Blanch the spinach leaves by boiling them in water for 1 minute. Then strain and rinse the spinach in cold water and gently squeeze out the excess water with your hands.

2 Place the blanched spinach in a large bowl and top with the remaining ingredients.

3 Mix together until the spinach is evenly coated in the sauce. Add more salt to taste if needed.

시금치 Sigumchi (spinach)

To many, spinach is considered a superfood, containing nutrients such as calcium, vitamins A, C, E, K1, folate, and magnesium. Spinach has been associated with eye, immune, and heart health among other things.

1 lb/455g spinach leaves

1 tbsp sesame oil

2 garlic cloves, minced

1 tbsp toasted sesame seeds

sea salt, to taste

Serves 2–4

숙주 Sukju Namul (bean sprout)

Bean sprouts contain vitamins C, K, manganese, phosphorus, and iron. They have been thought to enhance nutrient absorption, help alleviate anxiety, and improve bone and heart health.

1 lb/450g mung bean sprouts

1 tbsp sesame oil

1 tbsp sesame seeds

1 scallion (spring onion), finely chopped

sea salt and freshly ground black pepper, to taste

Serves 4

1 Blanch the mung bean sprouts by boiling them in water for 1 minute. Then strain and rinse the sprouts in cold water and gently squeeze out the excess water with your hands.

2 Place the blanched bean sprouts in a large bowl and top with the sesame oil, sesame seeds, and chopped scallion (spring onion).

3 Mix together until the bean sprouts are evenly coated in the sauce. Add salt and pepper to taste, if desired.

달래 Dallae (wild chive)

Spring is an exciting time for those who love the taste of Asian chives. This food is known to alleviate stomachaches and even help fight insomnia.

1 bunch/3–4oz/85–115g Asian chives, washed and dried, left whole

4 tbsp soy sauce

½ tbsp sesame oil

2 tbsp gochugaru (Korean red pepper flakes)

approx. 1 tbsp turbinado or white (caster) sugar (optional)

Serves 2–4

1 Remove the outer skin from the bulbs of the Korean wild chives.

2 In a large bowl, mix together the soy sauce, sesame oil, and gochugaru (red pepper flakes) with the Korean wild chives and leave to marinate for 30 minutes at room temperature. You can choose to add around 1 tablespoon of sugar to balance the flavor, but this is optional.

비빔밥 bibimbap

Bibimbap means "mixed rice," and is a simple, one-bowl dish that's both healthy and satisfying. Many Koreans eat bibimbap as a way to conveniently use up leftover rice and vegetables. Historically, bibimbap was consumed as a Lunar New Year's Eve dish to do just that—clear out any remaining food in preparation for a fresh start.

Bibimbap typically consists of rice topped with a few vegetables of various colors, along with some protein such as beef and a fried egg. The ingredients are mixed together with a hot pepper paste called gochujang (고추장), which transforms the various ingredients into one homogenous dish. The vegetables provide a diverse profile of nutrients and flavors. The protein, rice, oils, and sauce marry up with these vegetables to create a harmoniously delicious dish.

Like most other Korean dishes, bibimbap may be prepared in various ways depending on the region and time of year. Although bibimbap is typically known to contain cooked vegetables, it can also be made with fresh vegetables for a more light, summery taste.

simple bibimbap recipe

This basic bibimbap recipe makes for a quick yet delicious meal. Eat it with family or store it in a container to enjoy throughout the week.

3 cups/20oz/550g short-grain rice

1 large carrot, julienned

1 large red bell pepper (red pepper), thinly sliced

1 large zucchini (courgette), thinly sliced

1 large onion, thinly sliced

soy sauce, for seasoning

1lb/455g spinach leaves

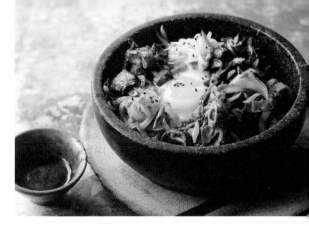

12oz/340g beef (ground or thinly sliced beef brisket) or protein of choice (seafood, tofu, etc.)

4 large eggs (1 per dish)

1–2 tablespoons gochujang (Korean red pepper paste) per bowl

toasted sesame seeds, for sprinkling (optional)

toasted sesame oil, for drizzling (optional)

2 scallions (spring onion), finely chopped

Serves 4

1 Cook the rice according to the packet instructions. While the rice is cooking, rinse and prepare the vegetables. Keep the vegetables separate and do not combine them.

2 Lightly grease a large pan with toasted sesame oil and place it on a medium heat. Sauté each vegetable except for the spinach, one by one, until they are lightly cooked but still a little crisp. You may add a dash of soy sauce to each vegetable to add flavor. Set the sautéed vegetables on one large dish in individual piles.

3 Use the recipe on page 58 to prepare the spinach.

4 Cook the beef or your choice of protein by sautéing it in a large pan until cooked through and set aside.

5 Fry the eggs sunny side up. One egg will be used per bowl.

6 Once all the ingredients are prepared, the bibimbap is ready to be served. Divide the cooked rice between four bowls, and top each one with a quarter of the beef or protein of your choice, and small amount of each vegetable. Place one fried egg on top. Add gochujang, and sprinkle with toasted sesame seeds and the chopped scallions (spring onion). You may add a drizzle of toasted sesame oil.

7 Once each bowl is prepared and served, each person can mix all the ingredients together and enjoy.

other healing dishes to try:

Luckily, the internet is chock full of amazing Korean recipes if you want to explore further—see page 136 for recommendations. Here are some other common healing dishes to try.

For hangovers:
해장국 Haejangguk (hangover soup)

Haejangguk refers to any type of soup that is consumed during a hangover. It most closely translates to "detox soup." Common ingredients for haejangguk include bean sprouts, cabbage, and ox blood. The bean sprouts contain a compound called asparagine, which theoretically lowers acetaldehyde, a byproduct of alcohol in the body that can influence hangover symptoms.

When you have belly issues:
죽 Juk (rice porridge)

Juk is a rice dish made by boiling rice for a long period of time, which allows the grains to expand and become creamy. In the old days, juk was commonly eaten by poor people who needed to stretch their food. Today, it is consumed to ease digestive burden or as a light meal, especially for breakfast. The flavor varieties of juk are endless, ranging from chicken and abalone (sea snails), to red bean and pumpkin.

When feeling under the weather:
설렁탕 Seolleongtang (ox-bone soup)

Ox bone soup is basically Korean bone broth. Ox bones are boiled for long periods to create a milky white broth rich in vitamins including A and K, minerals such as calcium, magnesium, and phosphorus and amino acids including proline and glycine. This soup is great for a cold winter's day, especially when you feel you need some extra nourishment.

For extra vitality: 콩국수 Kongguksu (noodles in cold soybean broth)

Kongkusu is a cold summer dish rich in protein. The broth is made with soybeans, which contain a number of beneficial nutrients including fiber, vitamin K, folate, copper, manganese, phosphorus, and calcium. Soybeans also contain a number of bioactive plant compounds including isoflavones, which act as an antioxidant in the body.

In the next chapter, you'll learn more about how Korean food is steeped in the country's culture and is one of the key tenets of Traditional Korean Medicine.

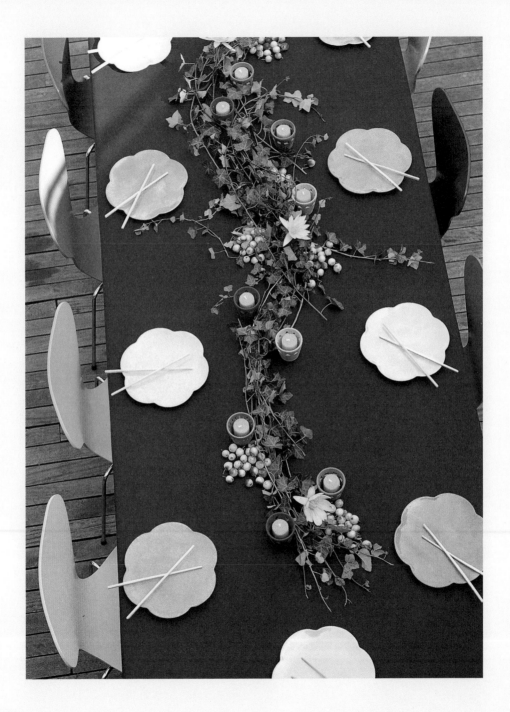

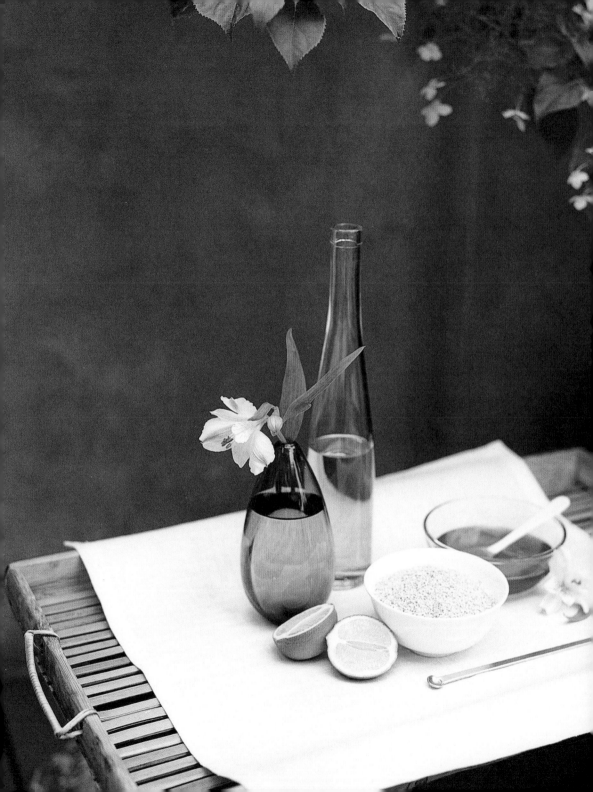

chapter 3

traditional korean medicine

I write this chapter as a curious consumer rather than a medical expert. Korean Medicine, or hanbang (한방) is a vast and specialized topic, which includes practices such as Saam acupuncture (traditional Korean acupuncture), moxibustion (medicine therapy involving burning mugworts on parts of the body), sasang typology (see page 68), and cupping (therapy involving heated suction on localized parts of the skin). However, I have chosen to focus on elements that you can incorporate into a self-care routine at home, such as food as medicine and herbal teas.

While the previous chapter covered some healing Korean foods, this chapter will dive deeper into their medicinal properties. It will also look at the underlying framework that has informed the evolution of the Korean way of life with regard to health. The philosophy of health and disease prevention is integrated into Korea's cultural norms, and these ideas may be applied to your everyday life as well.

Please consult with your healthcare practitioner before using any of the ideas in this chapter as treatments or alternative treatments for any conditions you may have, as this information is not meant to be construed as medical advice.

TKM vs TCM

Traditional Korean Medicine (TKM) has been influenced by Traditional Chinese Medicine (TCM), which is an alternative medical system that has evolved over thousands of years. Many would argue that TKM is rooted in TCM, and so they are not two completely distinctive schools of thought. However, TKM has transformed into its own distinctive practice that reflects Korea's unique culture, traditions, and regional differences. Likewise, TCM has evolved through centuries by reabsorbing the teachings of neighboring countries. As such, many of the elements of TCM and TKM are similar if not the same.

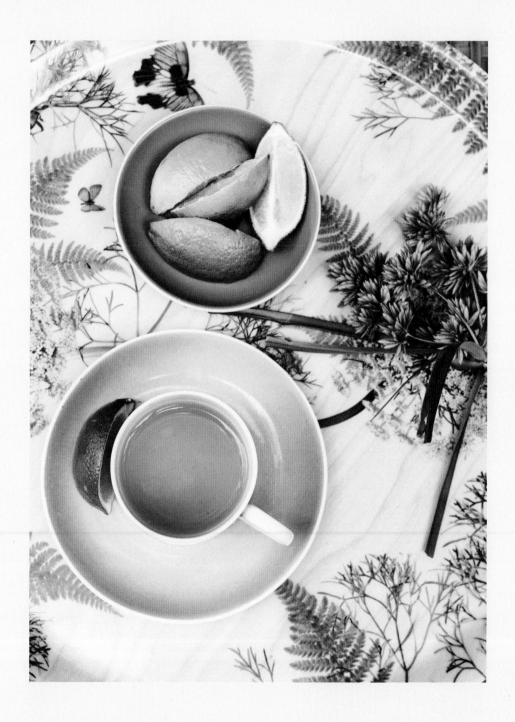

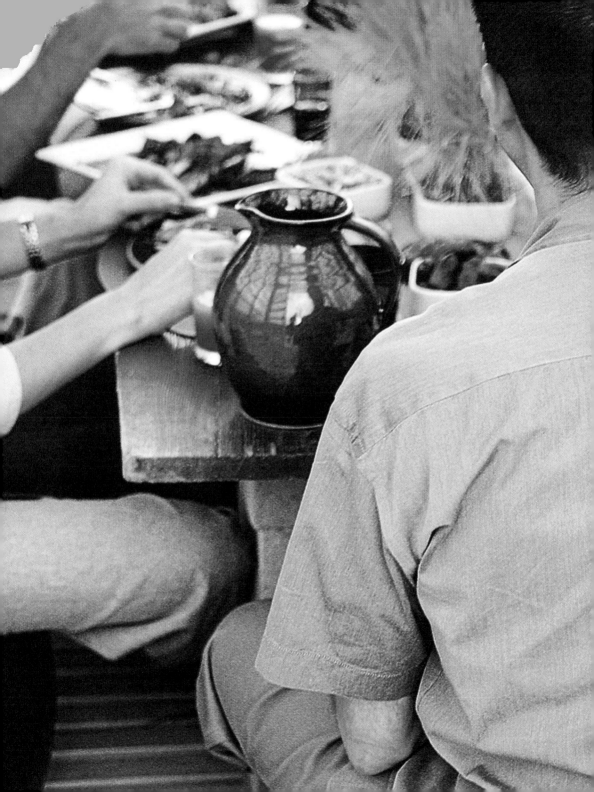

사상의학
sasang constitutional medicine

One of the main elements of TKM is Sasang typology, which categorizes individuals into four types based on their constitution. One's constitution is determined by anatomical and physiological traits. According to Sasang, an individual's biological type informs their personality, temperament, disease diagnosis, and treatment.

Below is a non-exhaustive list of traits for each of the four Sasang types:

Tae-eum: Heavy bones, thick waistline, higher body mass index, withdrawn, warm, adaptable, reflective, positive, prone to stroke and respiratory disease

So-Yang: Large spleen, small kidneys, inverted triangle body type, active, extroverted, impulsive, excitable, prone to kidney disease, high blood pressure, and depression

So-eum: Large kidneys, small spleen, balanced frame, introverted, cautious, negative, passive, prone to gastritis, stomach aches, and indigestion

Tae-Yang: Large lungs, small liver, large head, independent, charismatic, creative, prone to infertility, indigestion, and hip weakness

Although we may not be able to accurately assess our Sasang type without the help of a qualified practitioner, we can appreciate the personalized approach of constitutional medicine, which aims to take a person-centered rather than a symptom-centered approach to disease treatment.

이론의 5가지 요소
the five element theory

A foundational part of TKM stems from balancing yin and yang energies (see page 15) in the body. These energies are dictated by five complementary elements: wood, fire, earth, metal, and water. Each element is associated with its own season, organ systems in the body, taste profile, and color. The overarching philosophy of the five element theory is that all elements should be balanced, with no one element overpowering the rest.

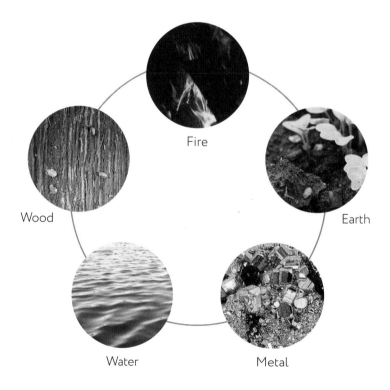

Fire

Wood

Earth

Water

Metal

Below is a brief representation of each element. Theoretically, the five tastes and types of food should be consumed in balance, which is what Korean cuisine aims to accomplish at its core.

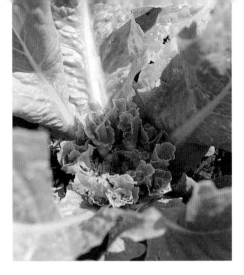

목재 Wood

Season: Spring

Associated organs: Gallbladder, liver, eyes, sinuses

Color: Green or blue

Taste profile: Sour

Sour foods exude a cooling quality and are used to treat conditions associated with excess fluidity such as diarrhea, over-perspiration, and sagging skin. This taste profile is also said to balance the mind and help organize scattered thoughts.

Sour food examples: Lemon, lime, sour plum, leek, vinegar

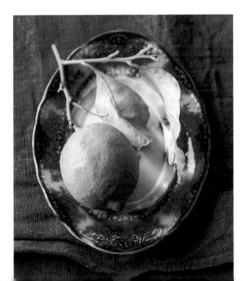

불 Fire

Season: Summer

Associated organs: Small intestine, heart, tongue, blood vessels

Color: Red

Taste profile: Bitter

Bitter flavors have a drying effect, helping to lower fevers, inflammation, and infection. They are said to clean arteries and alleviate conditions that are associated with dampness such as parasites, yeast overgrowth, skin conditions, and swellings. Lethargic and overweight individuals may benefit the most from bitter foods.

Examples of bitter foods: Romaine lettuce, alfalfa, rye, scallions (spring onions), vinegar

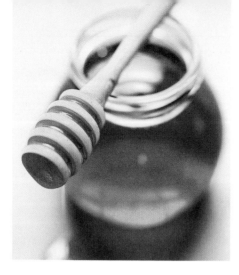

지구 Earth

Season: Late summer

Associated organs: Stomach, pancreas, mouth, muscles

Color: Yellow

Taste profile: Sweet

The sweet taste is known to harmonize other flavors and create a relaxing effect on the nervous system. It is said to be especially good for nervous individuals, as opposed to those who are sluggish or overweight.

Examples of sweet foods: Fruit, some vegetables, nuts and seeds, sweeteners such as honey

금속 Metal

Season: Fall

Associated organs: Large intestine, lungs, nose, skin

Color: White

Taste profile: Pungent

Foods of pungent and spicy flavor stimulate circulation and digestion. Pungent foods also disperse mucus throughout the body, thus clearing the lungs. Pungent flavors are beneficial for those feeling lethargic or sluggish. Many pungent herbs are said to be deeply warming, and therefore used to overcome feelings of coldness.

Examples of pungent foods: Cayenne, anise, dill, scallions (spring onions), cinnamon bark, cloves, rosemary, spearmint, basil, nutmeg, horseradish, ginger root

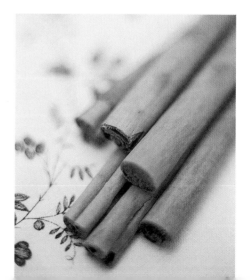

물 Water

Season: Winter

Associated organs: Bladder, kidneys, ears, bones

Color: Black

Taste profile: Salty

Foods with a salty flavor, when used properly, have a cooling and centering effect and are believed to improve digestion, detoxification, and concentration. Salt is also often used externally for sore throats and inflammation of the gums. Despite these benefits, salt should not be overconsumed and those with high blood pressure, edema, or lethargy should limit their intake.

Examples of salty foods: Seaweed, pickled foods, soy sauce

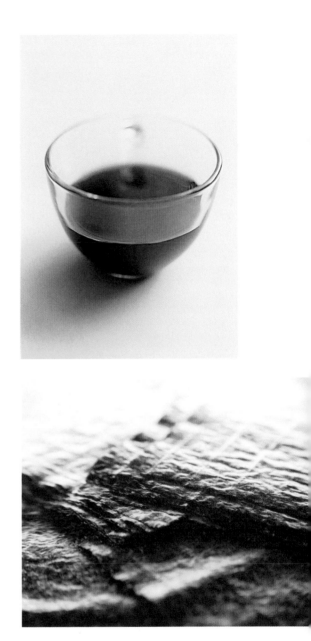

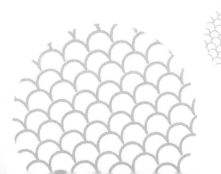

오방색 obangsaek

(the five color theory)

Complementary to the five element theory, obangsaek describes the five cardinal colors that correspond to each of the previously mentioned five elements. These colors are blue, red, yellow, black, and white. Getting your "5 a day" is an easy way to ensure that your meal contains variety and balances out the various organ systems of the body. Green is often substituted for blue when it comes to creating harmonious meals.

Below are some foods common in Korean cuisine that you may want to try fitting into your meals. For simplicity, you may try to consume a range of these colors regularly, although fitting each color into one meal is also great, as in the case of bibimbap (see page 60).

Blue/Green: Cucumber, zucchini (courgette), scallions (spring onions), wild sesame leaves

Red: Red beans, red peppers (fresh, dried, or powdered)

Yellow: Squash, sweet potatoes

Black: Black rice, black beans, and black sesame, as well as manna lichen, wood-ear mushroom, oak mushroom, seaweed

White: White rice, onion, garlic, potato, and lotus root.

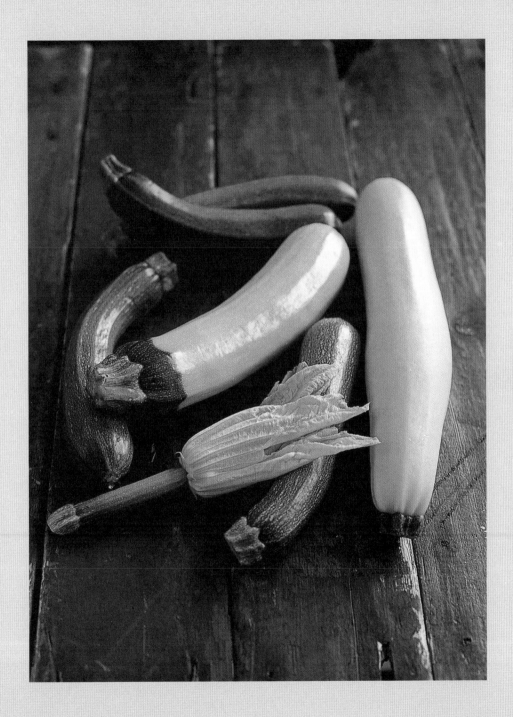

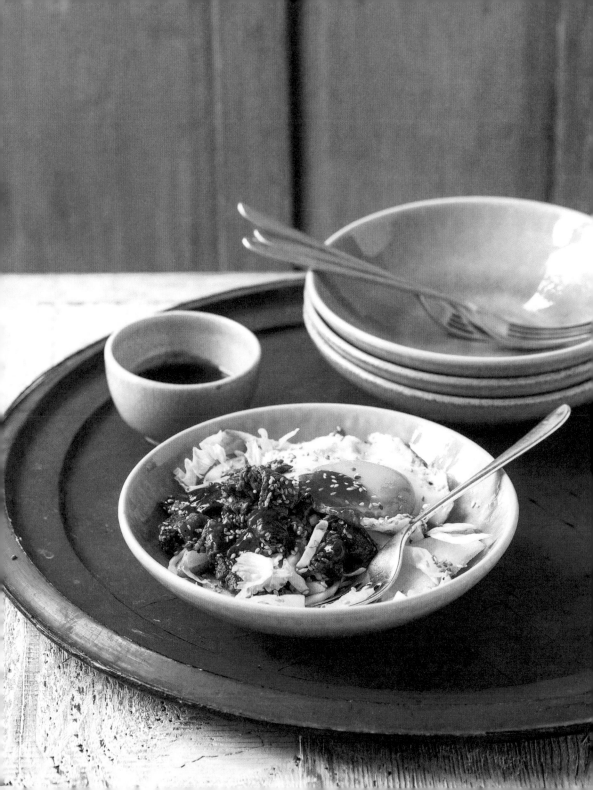

약식동원

yak sik dong won

(food and medicine are one)

I describe my beloved Korean food with three words: harmonious, balanced, and medicinal. The term yak sik dong won describes Korean gastronomy and roughly translates to "medicine and food share the same root." This belief points to food as the first line of defense against ill health—a frame of thought dating back centuries in Korea.

This philosophy of food within TKM does not simply mean reactively treating ailments with food as medicine, but also proactively strengthening the body's ability to heal itself. If the body is healthy and energized enough, it is better equipped to ward off disease. Korean food is about healing, but it's also about vitality.

Two terms capture the functional nature of food and herbs in TKM:

Boyangsik (보양식) or functional "energy food" to promote vitality and energy in one's life.

Boyak (보약) are supplemental and prescriptive herbal remedies used for disease prevention or to treat conditions, particularly ones demonstrating weakness or a lack of vitality.

As a nutritionist and wellness professional, I so appreciate the body's innate ability to heal itself. The philosophy of strengthening the body's healing mechanisms is something we can all practice. Even without a deep knowledge of TKM, we can be inspired by some of its general principles to keep our bodies healthy from the inside out.

Consume fermented foods

Fermented foods such as kimchi contain beneficial bacterial strains known as lactobacilli, which help to strengthen the immune system and protect against foodborne pathogens. Fermented foods other than kimchi include yogurts, kefir, and sauerkraut. Probiotic supplements may provide a similar benefit, although bio-individuality should be taken into account. This means that everyone's body has different needs. Getting advice from a nutritionist or other practitioner you trust may be a good idea.

Consume a high proportion of plant foods

Korean cuisine includes an abundance of vegetables and a colorful spectrum of ingredients. Colors from plant foods contain an array of phytonutrients, which keep the body healthy and compensate for the toxic load our bodies accumulate daily from factors such as pollutants, stress, food, and household products.

Consider your emotional wellbeing

Physician Lee Je-ma of the Joseon Dynasty (a dynastic kingdom lasting from 1392–1897 that shaped many of Korea's modern cultural norms) theorized that the health of the body is closely related to the mind, and that the state of someone's mental and emotional condition should be considered alongside bodily symptoms and environmental factors. The next two chapters provide further techniques to help nurture emotional wellbeing.

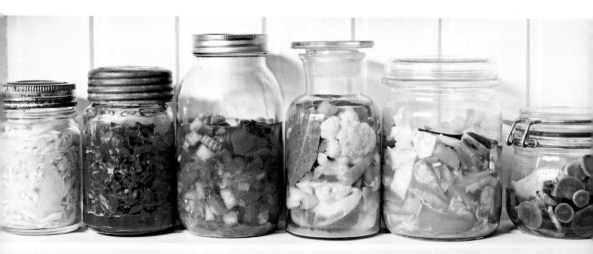

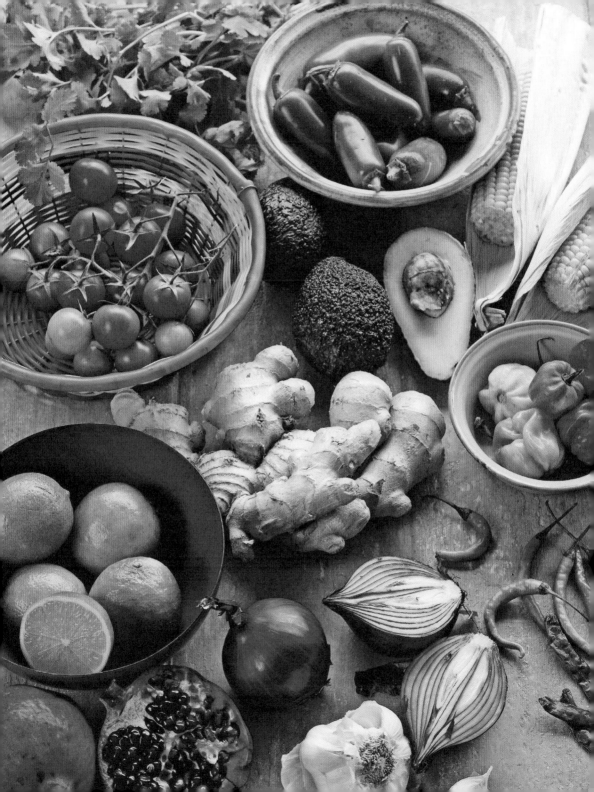

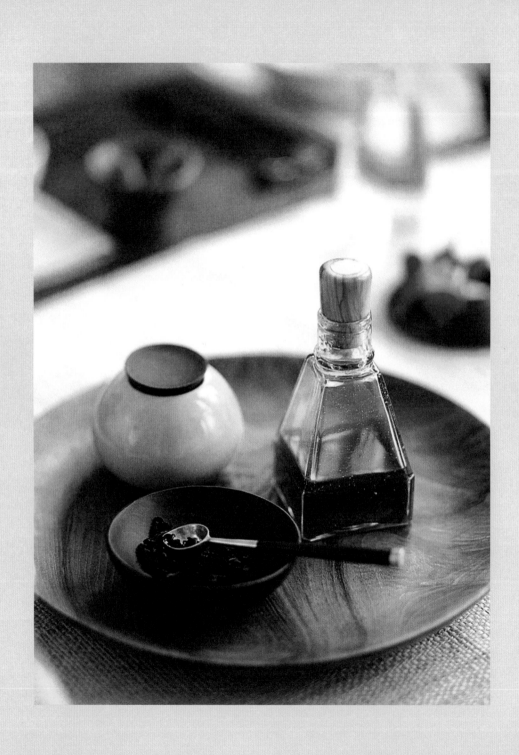

the three staple fermented sauces

More than just sauces, the items below represent foundational flavors in Korean cuisine, without which no Korean pantry is complete. What most people may not realize is that these sauces each offer medicinal benefits.

된장 Doenjang (soybean paste)

Made with fermented soybeans and salt, doenjang contains anti-inflammatory and antioxidant properties. It has also been shown to be beneficial to gut health by promoting the growth of friendly bacteria, which help our bodies digest food and absorb nutrients.

간장 Ganjang (soy sauce)

Soy sauce, especially salt-free or low-sodium varieties, may be protective against high blood pressure, cancer, and colitis. Soy sauce may also support healthy digestion and reduce allergic reactions.

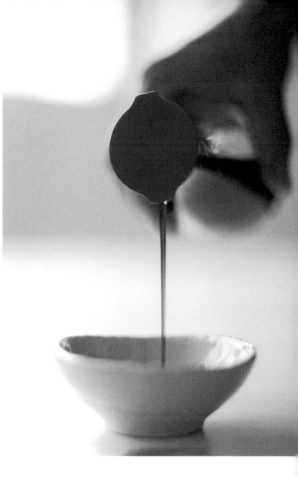

고추장 Gochujang (hot pepper paste)

Gochujang has been found to be beneficial for diabetes, by reducing insulin resistance (when cells in the body can't easily use glucose for energy). It is also beneficial for the prevention of cardiovascular disease as it helps reduce cholesterol levels.

healing herbs and ingredients

Herbalism, or the use of plants for their medicinal and therapeutic effects, is a key element in TKM. For example, *Poria cocos* (herbal mushroom) and *Polygala tenuifolia* (a type of root) may be used for the treatment of geonmang (건망), which refers to dementia, amnesia, or poor memory. Other plant materials such as cinnamon bark, licorice root, seaweed, and algae can also be used for various illnesses. I suggest that you consult with your doctor before using herbs or extracts. You could also get advice from a qualified herbalist.

One of the more popular plants is ginseng, or insam (인삼), which is used in Korea for a variety of therapeutic effects. Ginseng is a potent antioxidant and used to treat conditions such as brain fog, diabetes, digestive and respiratory disorders, and erectile dysfunction. You may have noticed that it is a staple ingredient in the Samgyetang soup on page 54.

Another example is raw garlic, or maneul (마늘), which is found in most Korean sauces. Also known as yangnyom (양념), it is used to aid digestion and cleanse the blood by theoretically optimizing the kidney and livers' ability to filter out waste and toxins. Garlic is also known to boost the immune system and help reduce cholesterol.

Other healing ingredients include:

생 감자 주스 Raw potato juice: Used to soothe the stomach due to its alkaline effect, which balances out acidity

개암 Gaeam (hazelnut): Used for skin health, includes vitamins and minerals that are beneficial for pregnant women

황태 Hwangtae (dried pollock fish): Believed to help the body regain energy

막걸리 Makgeolli: A light rice wine typically made from rice or barley containing potential anticancer and antioxidant properties

김 Gim (dried edible seaweed): Rich in iodine for thyroid function, contains anti-inflammatory properties

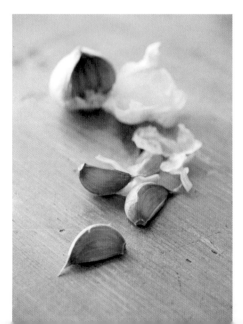

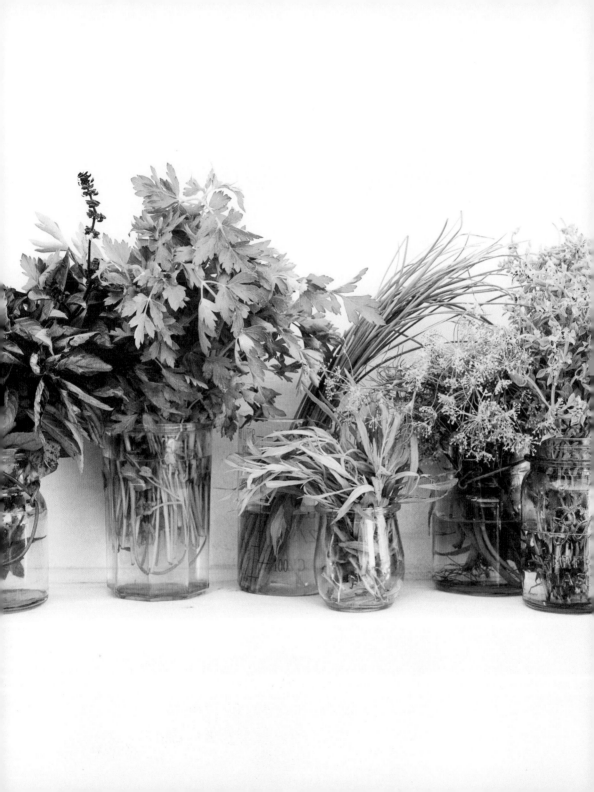

korean herbal teas

Consuming medicinal tea is very much a part of Korean culture. In fact, the practice of Korean traditional tea ceremonies, or darye (다례), can be traced back to around as early as 18 B.C. Tea was always consumed in my household when I was growing up and added a post-dinner closure to the day. It wasn't until recently that I learned about the various health-giving qualities of Korean herbal teas, and their digestive benefits especially after a meal.

These are some of my favorite Korean teas. Many of them can be found in a Korean grocery store, while some can be made from scratch at home.

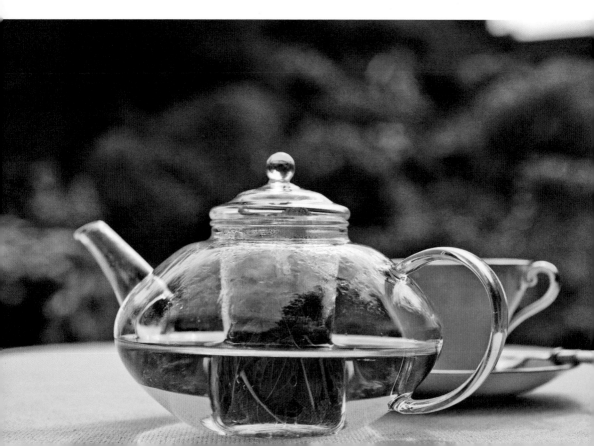

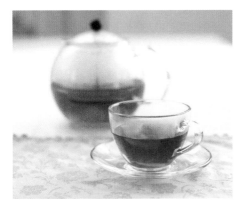

녹차 Nogcha (green tea)

Nogcha, or green tea, is rich in antioxidants and anti-inflammatory compounds known as polyphenols. These provide a variety of benefits including improved fat burning, brain function, and cardiovascular health.

How to make:
Use green tea bags or powdered matcha and prepare according to the packet instructions.

생강차 Saenggang-cha (ginger tea)

Saenggang-cha is a simple ginger tea that can help alleviate several ailments such as nausea, the common cold, and digestive issues. It is also known to lower blood pressure, reduce inflammation, and soothe heartburn.

How to make (1 serving):
There are many ways to make ginger tea, but here is a simple method. Wash and peel a 1-in (2.5-cm) piece of fresh ginger and thinly slice it into a mug. Pour in 1–1½ cups/8–12fl oz/225–350ml boiling water and allow to steep for 3–5 minutes. If you wish, you may add a cinnamon stick, 1 tsp of honey, and a few pine nuts.

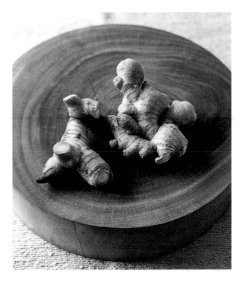

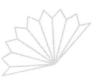

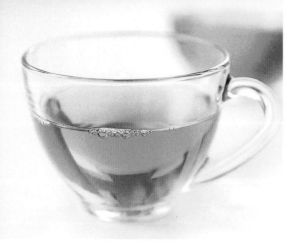

대추차 Daechu-cha (jujube tea)

Daechu-cha is made with jujubes (see page 54), and is a popular drink for combating constipation, while boosting the immune system as well as circulation. Jujubes are high in vitamin C and other antioxidants, and are thought to calm the mind by reducing anxiety. The phenolic compounds found in jujubes also make this tea rejuvenating for the skin and aid sleep.

How to make (6–8 servings):
Wash 6–8 dried jujubes or red dates and slice in half. Place the jujubes in a pot with 6–8 cups/48–64fl oz/1.4–1.9 litres of boiling water along with a 1-in (2.5-cm) piece of peeled and sliced fresh ginger and a cinnamon stick. You may also add honey to taste if you prefer a sweeter flavor. Boil for 30 minutes and strain the liquid before serving. Top the tea with a few pine nuts.

율무차 Yulmu-cha ("Job's tears" tea)

Yulmu-cha is a unique drink that is quite different from other teas you may have tried. It is made from powdered Job's tears and sometimes nuts, making it a thick, hearty, and creamy drink rich in protein and fat. The star ingredient of this drink is Job's tears—a grain plant known to fight cholesterol, arthritis, and respiratory tract infections among other ailments.

How to make (1–2 servings):
Acquire a bag of Job's tears and blitz them into a powder in a food processor. In a pot, simmer 3 tbsp of the powder with 2 cups/17fl oz/500ml of water for 30 minutes. If you wish, you may add a dash of milk or alternative milk and add 1–2 tbsp honey to taste. Store the remaining powdered Job's tears in a sealed bag or container at room temperature, or in the refrigerator for maximum freshness.

보리차 Boricha (barley tea)

Boricha is perhaps the most commonly consumed tea in Korea. Made with roasted barley, it is sometimes drunk in place of water, and many Korean households have a pitcher of barley tea in their refrigerator. Boricha acts as a natural antacid, alleviating heartburn and acid reflux. It is high in vitamin C, which strengthens immunity and lowers inflammation. Barley is rich in Gamma aminobutyric acid (GABA), a neurotransmitter or chemical messenger in the brain that helps you unwind.

How to make (2–4 servings):
Acquire roasted pearl barley grains online or from a Korean or Asian food store. Boil 1 tbsp of the grains with 4 cups/30fl oz/900ml of water for 5 minutes. Serve and enjoy either hot or cold. You can also store this in the fridge for up to five days.

메밀차 Memil-cha (buckwheat tea)

One of my favorite post-dinner teas, memil-cha improves circulation and contains various antioxidants including vitamin E, which is known to boost immunity by combatting free radicals (unstable, potentially damaging molecules) in the body. It also aids digestion by alleviating bloating and constipation, and contains compounds that may help reduce the risk of cancer.

How to make (2 servings):
You can buy roasted buckwheat grains from your local Korean or Asian grocery. Steep 2 tbsp of the grains in 3 cups/24fl oz/700ml of water for 3–5 minutes.

other teas to try

The following teas are a bit harder and less economical to make from scratch, but they are readily available either online or in your local Korean or Asian grocery.

유자차 Yuja-cha (honey-citron tea)

This tea is often served as a remedy for the common cold due to its high vitamin C content. It also contains honey, which helps soothe the throat. Yuja-cha mix is usually sold in jars and has a syrup-like consistency.

매실차 Maesil-cha (plum tea)

Maesil-cha is made with Korean plums. A popular drink, it is known to help with detoxification and fatigue. Therefore, it is often served after a large meal. This tea can be made by purchasing Korean plum extract and mixing in 2 tbsp of extract with every ½ cup/4fl oz/120ml of water along with a few ice cubes.

둥글레차 Doongulae cha (Solomon's seal tea)

Doongulae cha is a soothing tea with a roasted and nutty taste made from the dried ground root of a Solomon's seal plant. As with many of the other teas listed, it is often served after a meal for its digestive benefits. It is also soothing to the throat and lungs, and used to treat some skin conditions. The easiest way to make this tea is by acquiring tea bags.

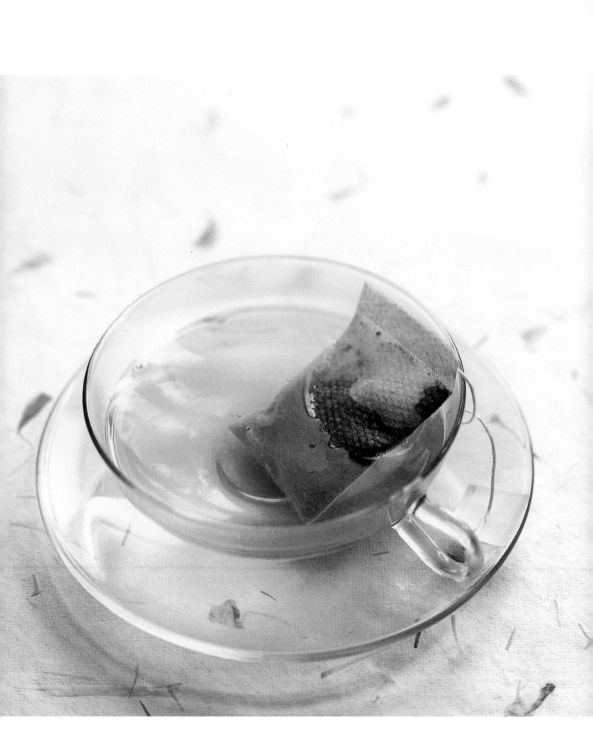

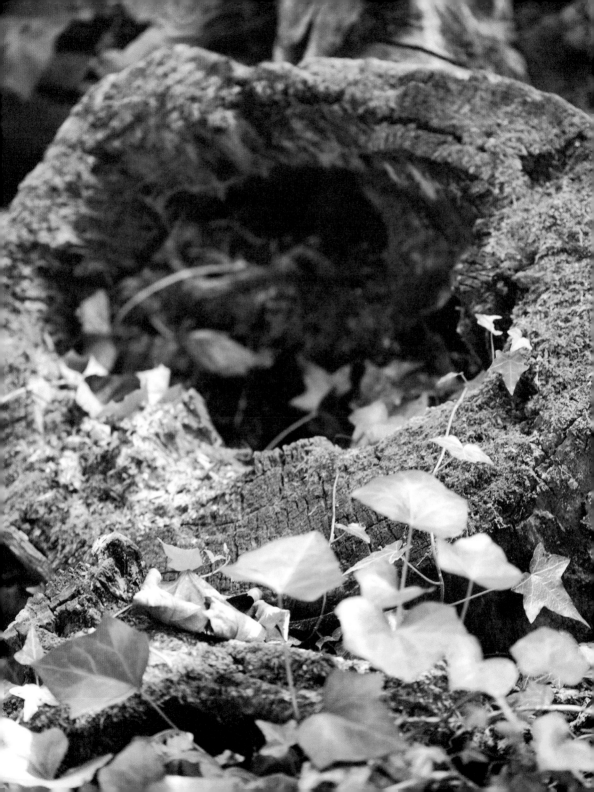

nature and forest

In 2012, halfway through my time living in Korea, I remember feeling sad and morose. It was fall, and the shift in the weather from warm to cold represented to me the dawn of a new year; a transition from old to new. This step into the unknown can feel unsettling, and for some reason, it hit me especially hard that year as I was in the process of navigating difficult emotions and circumstances.

I remember one weekend deciding to take a solo trip to Nami Island, a river island in the North Han River. Nami island is a beautiful destination even on an alright day, but in the fall, the tall, perfectly aligned trees adorned with multicolored foliage make it almost fairy-tale-like. As I set foot on the island after a long train ride and a ferry trip, I immediately smelled the depth of the forest and felt gratitude and peace.

A welcome escape from my melancholy thoughts, I observed children, families, adults, and elders bask in the golden rays of the sun while laughing, eating, playing, and walking as if no day could ever be better than this one.

I don't know what it was, but on that day, the forest healed me.

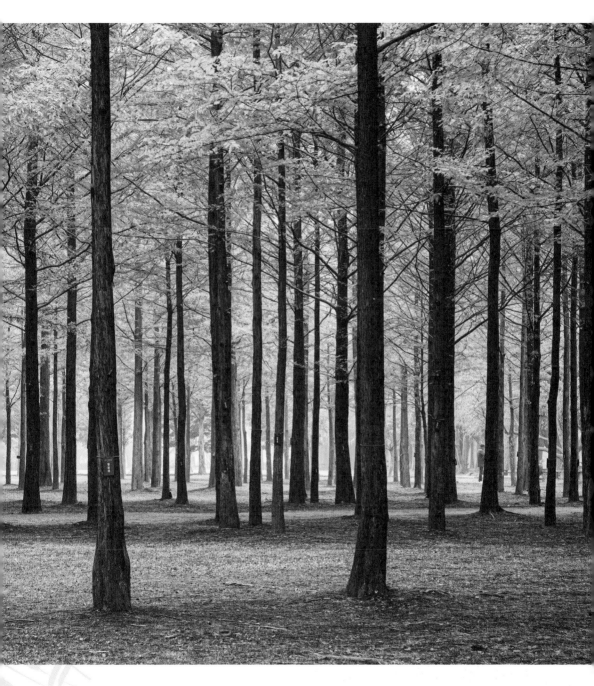

살림욕 salim yok

(forest bathing)

There is a universal truth to the idea that the forest can heal.
There is something about immersing yourself in natural
surroundings that can ground you and make you feel innately
human. Nature's ability to give us a sense of peace is
increasingly recognized, especially in Korea, where the
government has acknowledged nature as a cultural collective
value and invested in forest managment and welfare programs.

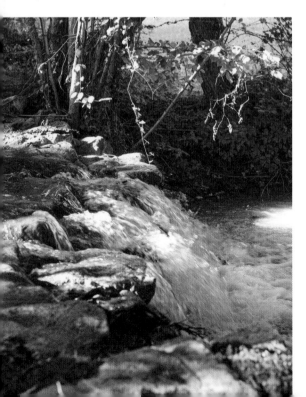

A direct translation of the Japanese concept of shihrin yoku, salim yok, or forest bathing, is the act of spending time in a forest to reap its many healing benefits. The Korean government recognizes this concept as a welfare-promoting practice and actively invests millions of dollars into nature therapy programs. In fact, the Korean government has been designating a growing number of areas as "healing forests" with forest healing instructors, who facilitate guided walks and mindful activities in the forest to promote mind–body healing.

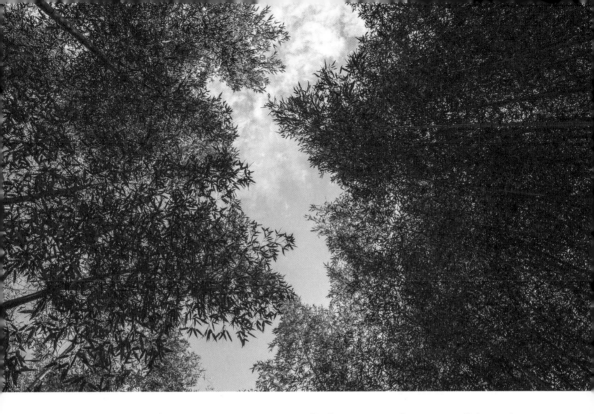

Forest bathing has become so renowned that it is now referred to as a medicinal practice, and the body of research around it continues to grow. According to studies by Dr. Qing Li, the Chairman of the Japanese Society of Forest Medicine, forest bathing has many benefits, including:

• **Lowering blood pressure:** Salim yok has been shown to reduce blood pressure and have protective benefits against heart disease.

• **Stimulating the parasympathetic nervous system:** Spending time in nature stimulates the "rest and digest" nervous system that functions to calm, relax, and improve sleep quality.

• **Reducing stress hormones:** Salim yok may reduce stress hormones such as cortisol and adrenaline, steering you away from the "fight or flight" state.

• **Immunity and anticancer effects:** Forest bathing has been found to be a form of preventative medicine, increasing the activity of natural "killer" cells, which can help control infections, defend against tumors, and boost levels of anti-cancer proteins.

• **Boosting mental health:** Salim yok may reduce anger and symptoms of depression and anxiety, while increasing mental clarity.

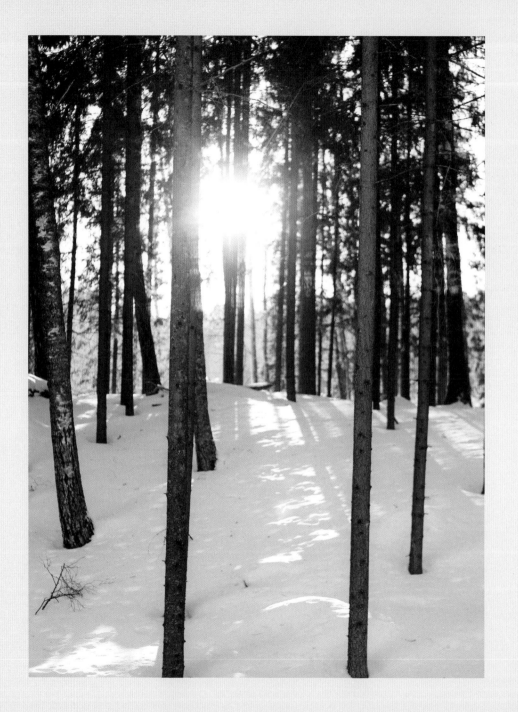

experience nature with your senses

Try practicing forest bathing yourself by going to a forest, wooded area, or other natural area and following these prompts.

1 Hear

Listen to the wind rustle the leaves and branches. Hear the birds singing and the soothing sound of a running stream if there's one nearby.

2 Smell

Notice the scent of the trees or the distinct smell in the air as the seasons change. Stop to smell the flowers or foliage.

3 Touch

Feel the texture of different stones and rocks. Touch the bark of a tree and notice a blade of grass grazing your leg.

4 Taste

Taste the fresh air.

5 See

Observe the rays of the sun cutting through the trees. Notice both the imperfect and precise shapes in nature. Find as many naturally occurring colors as possible such as reds, greens, browns, and yellows.

nature across the lifespan

The healing effects of the forest may be experienced and enjoyed by individuals of any age, including babies, children, adolescents, adults, and senior citizens. For teenagers, the forest may be a therapeutic outlet for feelings of angst and aggression and a source of inspiration for creativity. For adults, the forest may be an escape from burnout and stress while for elders, the forest can provide a relief from depressive thoughts. For individuals of all ages, it can be a detox from our perpetual reliance on technology.

my friend Gian

We can read about many Korean concepts online, but my favorite way to truly grasp the depth of Korean traditions is through my or someone else's unique lived experience.

My dear friend Gian Petersen is a shining example of someone who has stayed true to her roots and embraced nature and the forest in her own life. Born in 1939, Gian grew up in South Korea in the 1940s and became a Republic of Korea Army Nurse before immigrating to the United States, where I was fortunate enough to cross paths with her decades later.

When I ask Gian about her upbringing, she recounts that as Korea is a mountainous peninsula surrounded by the sea, she did not know anything different to loving and embracing nature as the foundation of her life. Many trees were chopped down as a consequence of the Korean War between North and South Korea from 1950–1953, so she and her classmates planted trees every year from elementary school until college during Sikmogil (식목일), an annual national celebration on April 5 created to promote and appreciate nature. Arable areas were such a commodity in Korea that every patch of available land in her childhood home was used to grow

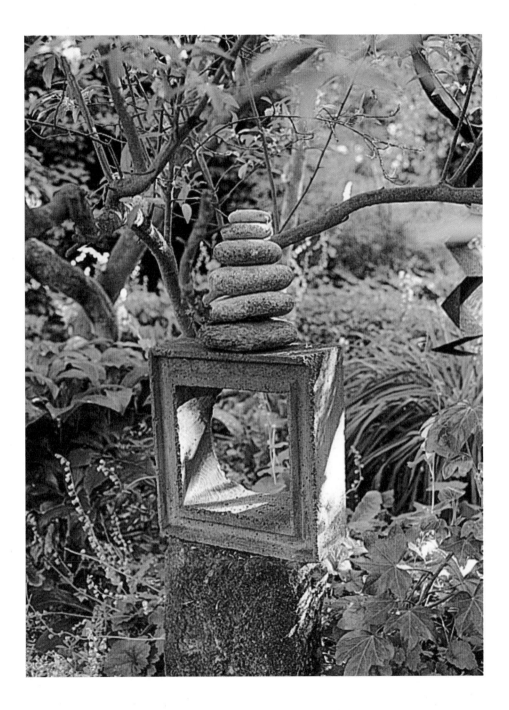

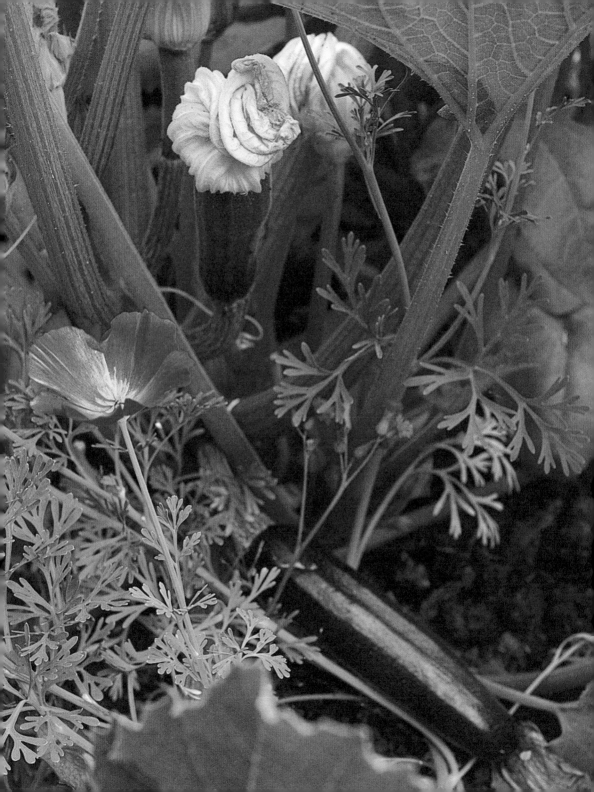

vegetables, and there was little space to play outside.

During her days as an army officer, Gian adoringly remembers camping out in the forest in Korea and enjoying the sights, sounds, and smells of her natural surroundings. She vividly remembers bathing in the mountains and cooking among the trees.

About 20 years ago, Gian invested in a 7-acre plot of historical land in the city of Virginia Beach, Virginia, and she recalls planting Korean gingko, persimmon, and chestnut trees along with a variety of flowers and plants before even settling into her new home. Gian had a vision that most people do not: that nature is not an optional accessory, but a necessary complement to our very existence. Because of her long-term patience, she now lives off the fruit, nuts, and plants that her land abundantly provides for her daily. She harvests her own honey, which she adds to her Korean plum tea, and makes side dishes with her edible grasses.

Gian's enthusiasm for sharing traditional Korean practices with others has led her to start preparing her land to become a teaching ground for others who want to learn about Korean farming practices. In her old age, Gian's one wish is to pass down her knowledge and appreciation of nature to younger generations.

Gian's advice is this:

Practice gratitude for all living things

According to Gian, we are all connected, whether with trees or with weeds. We are never alone because our natural surroundings are not separate from us, but part of us.

Cultivate positivity and creativity from nature

Every morning, Gian wakes up and sits outside among her plants and trees to take in the calmness of nature, allowing her mind to become still. This is where her greatest ideas come from.

Spend ample time in nature

A significant majority of the Korean population spends time in nature, whether it be through hiking or simply walking. According to Gian, nature is one of the greatest sources of peace and we should take advantage of nature's free offering as much as possible.

hiking culture

One of my fondest memories from living in Korea is hiking up a mountain called Bukhansan—a national treasure located in Seoul. The 4–5 hour uphill hike through the forest is a challenge for the average individual, but the hardest part is the last stretch, where you are at almost 45 degrees, holding on to thick cables to make it to the pointy peak of the mountain. Once you spot the cables, you know you are near the end and proud of your hard work, but it's what you see next that humbles you to your core. One by one, Korean senior citizens are on their way down the steep hill, proving to be avid hikers even into their old age.

In Korea, hiking is not just a pastime, but a cultural staple. A significant portion of Korean citizens venture out on a hike more than once a month to enjoy the therapeutic effects of the great outdoors and to escape the pressures of everyday life. A whopping 80 percent of Koreans visit a forest at least once a year. When hiking in Korea, you will often notice families and groups equipped with thoughtfully packed meals, picnicking along the trail. Eating along the mountain path is the highlight of most hikers' journeys, and a welcome respite from the hustle and bustle of the city.

What we can learn from Korean hiking culture:

Appreciate the marvels of your natural surroundings, no matter how familiar they are to you
The inspiring thing about Korean hikers is they don't lose appreciation of their nearby destinations. It can be easy to forget that even the natural wonders closest to you should not be taken for granted. Watching Korean hikers is almost like watching tourists discovering faraway land. Their appreciation for nature is palpable, and their exploratory spirit is contagious.

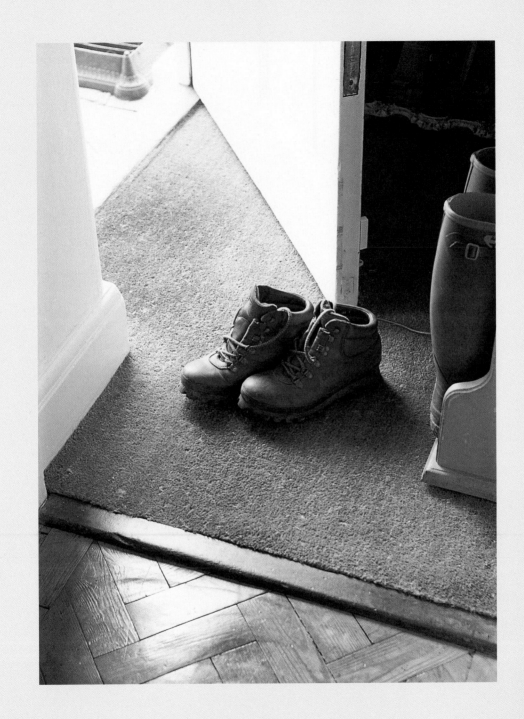

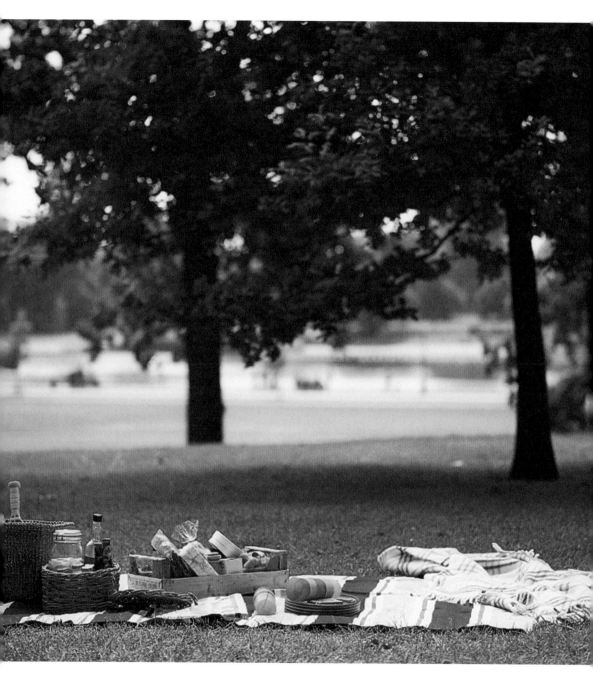

Pack your meal with thought and care

There is something about eating a meal in the middle of a nature path far from home, with no alternative access to sustenance, that makes you feel a newfound gratitude for food. As such, picnicking in the mountains is an experience that warms the spirit and comforts the soul.

Bring a friend, or a few

In Korea, hiking is very much a familial or a communal activity. Of course, hiking solo can bring great peace, but hiking with others reminds you that solitude and companionship don't have to be mutually exclusive.

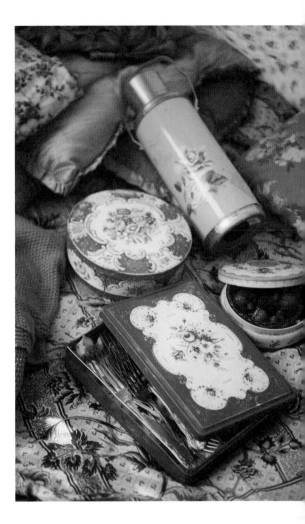

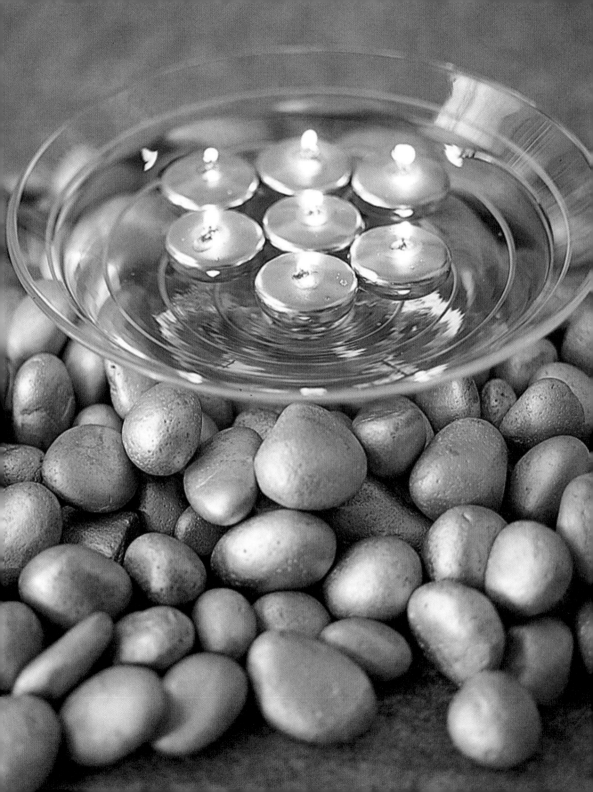

chapter 5

mindfulness and relaxation

A few years after I left Korea, I sat with a group of strangers in a yoga teacher training class. It was our first day, so we took turns going around in a circle to introduce ourselves and explain why we had decided to attend. One girl casually talked about her ongoing struggle with depression and anxiety. I was taken aback by how she could dare to be so vulnerable to share this information publicly. I related to her privately and silently while admiring her bravery.

Common mental disorders continue to be slowly destigmatized. Korea did not strike me as a place where mental health was a collective priority when I lived there from 2011–2013. Unfortunately, stress and depression have been a silent crisis in Korea for many years. It has been reported that nearly 75 percent of Korean elders suggest that mental health disorders such as depression are a sign of weakness.

Fortunately, the world has made leaps and strides towards normalizing and acknowledging chronic stress, burnout, and other factors that threaten mental well-being. Mental health has become a value of our generational youth. This is especially important in Korea where a stressful lifestyle affects so many.

On the following pages are some concepts and terms that have gained popularity in Korea relatively recently.

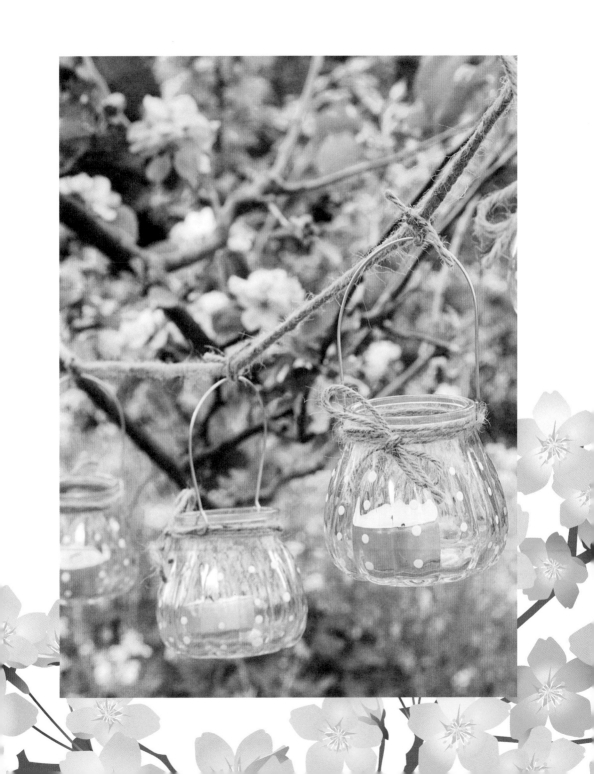

소확행 sohwakhaeng

(small but certain happiness)

Korea's younger generations are constantly churning out new slang terms, usually ones that merge shorter words or parts of other words to make a new one. One such term is sohwakhaeng, which literally translates to small (소 so) but certain (확 hwakh) happiness (행 haeng).

Although this concept may seem to be steeped in traditional wisdom, it was actually created and popularized by the pop-group sensation BTS in 2018 to convey freedom from worry about the future or appearances.

Maybe it's that first-sip-of-coffee feeling, the joy of holding and reading a hardcover book, or the sight of your dog's tail wagging joyously. All of these moments add up to help us live to see another day amidst an uncertain future.

Here are some ideas for how to practice sohwakhaeng in your own life:

1 Make a list of small and simple pleasures that you experience in everyday life. Many times, you can find pleasure within the familiarity and predictability of daily rituals: your bedtime routine, changing out of your work clothes for the day, or taking your first bite of breakfast.

2 Try your best to focus on things that are free. With the rise of consumerism, it's easy to get swept up in the belief that you need to spend money in order to feel pleasure. Instead, focus on things that appeal to your five senses: sights, sounds, feelings, tastes, and smells.

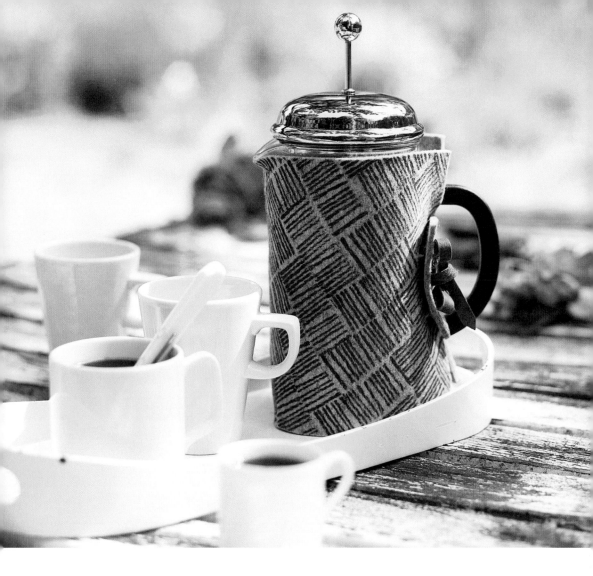

3 Stay present in your day and be mindful of as many small satisfying moments as possible. When we believe that every day brings simple pleasures, however small, we can rest assured that we don't have to wait for some distant future to feel content.

4 Finally, try your best to take your mind off the uncertain future. Dwelling on things beyond our control only brings pain. Remember that life always is, and will forever be, today.

멍때리기

hitting mung

A newer concept in Korea, hitting mung is the art of spacing out, or reaching a state of mung (멍), which means blankness, or the notion of being zoned out. It's no surprise that this has become a wellness trend in Korea, especially in the city, where the buzzing, chaotic, fast-paced energy has many living a high-stakes and high-stress lifestyle.

Although this concept may seem similar to meditation, it's actually fundamentally different. While meditation is process-driven and is a means to a long-term transformation, hitting mung is meant to provide an immediate and temporary dose of quiet. It's the act of pausing the mind. The journey to achieving a state of mung can come in many forms—sitting in nature, staring off into space, or staring at a wall or even at fire.

The informal nature of hitting mung makes it less of a practice and more of a simple tool that can be accessed from anywhere and at any time.

The popularity of hitting mung has bred spin-offs of the concept:

숲멍 forest mung

Spacing out while looking at or imagining trees, foliage, or other naturally occurring wonders of the forest.

불멍 fire mung

Spacing out while staring at or imagining burning flames, a fireplace, or a campfire.

물멍 **water mung**

Spacing out while staring at or
imagining any body of water:
a stream, a river, or the ocean.

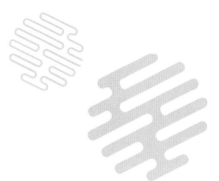

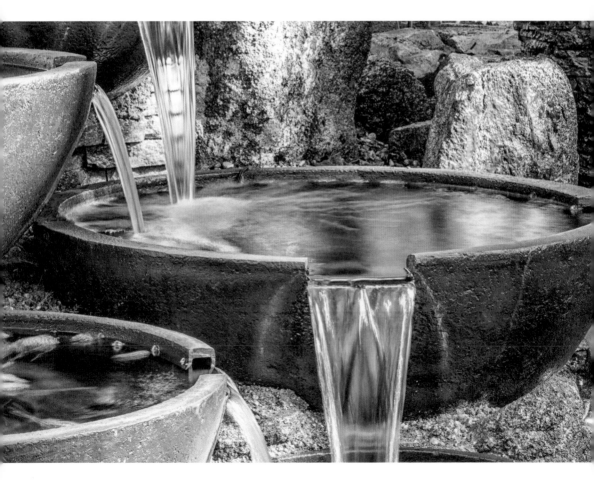

how to hit your own mung

1 The first thing to keep in mind is to not overthink the how. Just let your mind go blank—you can hit mung right now, as you are.

2 When you close your eyes and think of a natural scene that brings you peace, what comes to mind? Whether it's a body of water, a forest, or a mountain, print out a picture of that scene and keep it at your desk. If you can see this just by looking out of your window, even better!

3 When you feel your stress elevating or you just need a break, stare at this scene for several minutes and zone out.

4 Remember that hitting mung can come in any form. Make this your very own personal practice. Your happy place is your healing space.

5 Don't know where to start? Just stare at the wall.

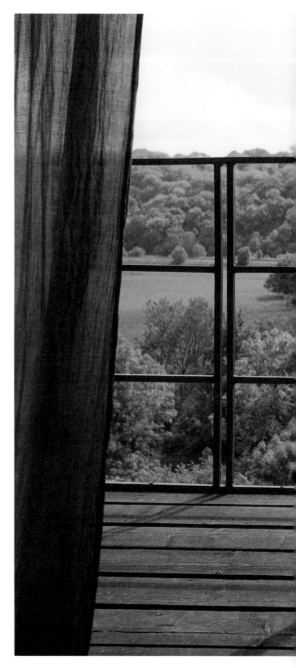

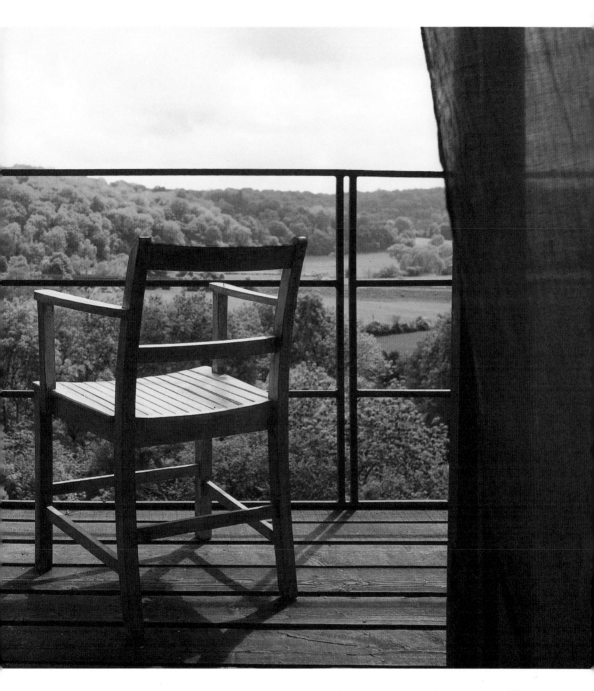

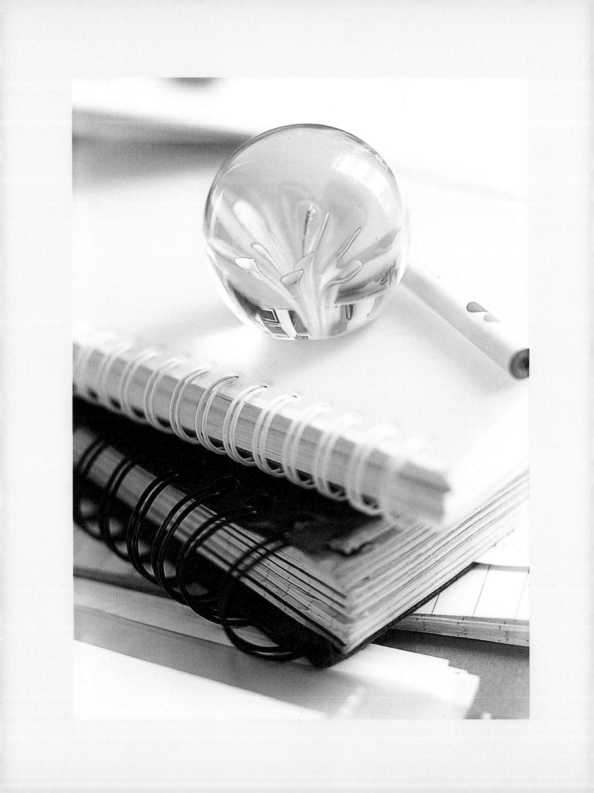

워라블 worabel

(work—life balance)

Coined by the younger generation, worabel is a slang term meaning "work–life" balance. This new term appropriately comes at a time when attitudes towards work are slowly evolving in response to the rising rate of unemployment, depression, exceedingly long work weeks, and high societal expectations—all of which have been lowering Koreans' quality of life for decades. The solution? Valuing boundaries between work and life, and prioritizing self-care over a higher salary.

practicing worabel in your own life

· Schedule self-care time just as you would a work meeting. Whether it be exercising, cooking a healthy meal, taking a bath to decompress, or connecting with a friend, practice taking care of yourself like it's your job—because it is.

· Define what setting boundaries between work and life means to you. For some, it's having a set transition time between work and free time, while for others it can mean a blended day of work with personal time sprinkled in throughout.

· When you're not at work, consider brain dumping any work-related anxieties that come to you in a journal to address later. This way, you can practice being present instead of mentally preoccupied.

· Continuously strive to reach your own state of unique equilibrium and harmony between life and work. There are no rules to worabel—as long as you are doing what makes you happy in the end.

묵상 meditation

The idea of meditation is nothing new in Korea, especially since about a quarter of the population is considered Buddhist, and meditation is a key part of Buddhism. Contrary to the concept of hitting mung, which allows the mind to wander freely, meditation is a more intentional practice of guiding the mind to a destination in pursuit of internal transformation, even if that destination is nothingness.

Meditation is considered a simple way to reduce and manage stress, increase self-awareness, focus on the present, and reduce negative thoughts. It may be especially beneficial to those who suffer from anxiety, asthma, depression, high blood pressure, and sleep issues. For many, it could be considered one of the most accessible forms of self-care, since everything you need to conduct meditation is already within you.

On the following pages you'll find several types of meditations that have their origins or roots in Korea. Although they vary, I would say they all share the overlapping tenet of increasing mindfulness and drawing focus inward rather outward. Look at them as tools, and less as ideologies.

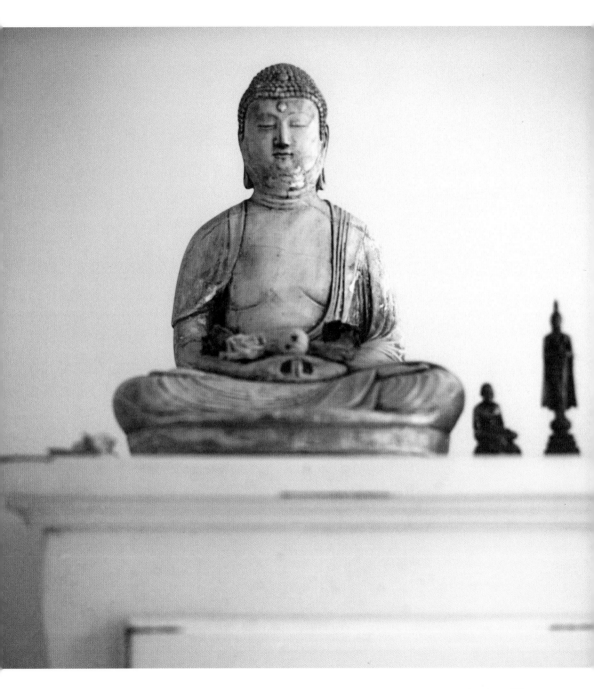

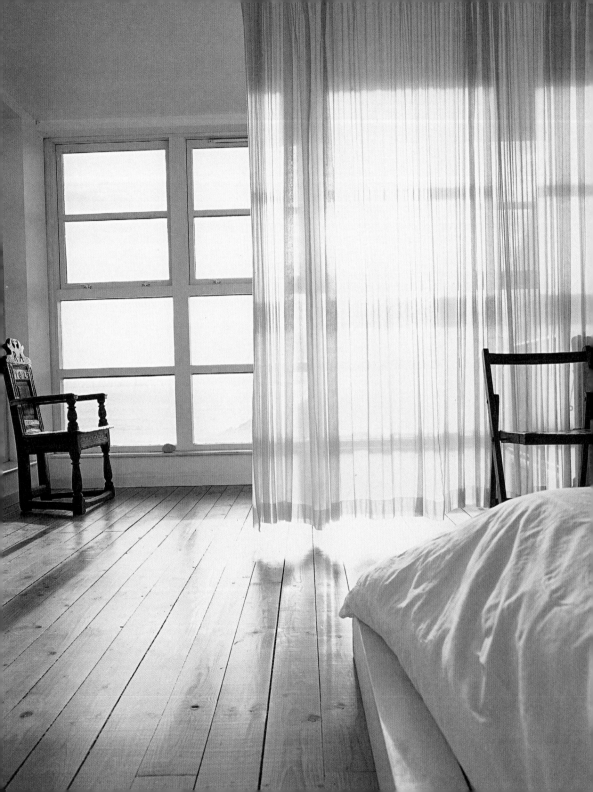

마음 수련 **maum su-ryun (mind training) meditation**

Maum su-ryun meditation is a technique to separate the "false" mind from reality, suggesting a distinction between the mind and consciousness. It was founded relatively recently, in 1996 by Woo Myung, a spiritual teacher who once said "It is my hope that all people in this world will discard themselves and live as complete people."

By diminishing the "false" mind, one is thought to expand their consciousness and in essence, become complete, discover one's true self, and find eternal happiness. Maum Su-ryun benefits the individual by allowing them to adopt a universal mind and as such, live for others toward the collective achievement of world peace. It is a twofold approach: to discard the old mind, and to attain a new one.

Since its inception in 1996, Maum su-ryun has expanded to over 300 centers in nearly 40 countries. It is safe to say that this and the following forms of meditation take time, commitment, and patience to master. However, you can still feel its benefits by trying this system out as a casual beginner.

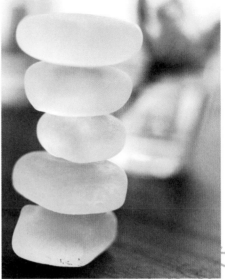

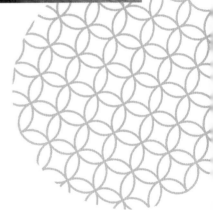

국선도 kouk sundo breathing

Kouk Sundo, or Sundo for short, is a form of meditation rooted in Taoism, a philosophical school of thought that revolves around living in harmony with Tao, which is defined as the natural order of the universe. To some, Sundo can be considered not only a form of meditation, but a complete technique that involves breathing and moving through the body's meridians to stimulate Ki, or internal energy.

The meditation portion of a Sundo practice involves a combination of holding anywhere from 1 to 25 postures while conducting rhythmic abdominal breathing to stimulate the Theta brainwave state. Postures are adjusted with skill level. One of the long-term aims of Sundo meditation is to synchronize the breath to our various organ systems and create overall "coherence" within the body.

The practice of Sundo entails three phases, the first of which flows through light stretches that prepare the body and joints for deep breathing and energetic circulation. The second phase involves sustained breathing, posture holds, and mental focus. The last phase involves more enlivening stretches and exercises aimed at spreading Ki energy to various parts of the body.

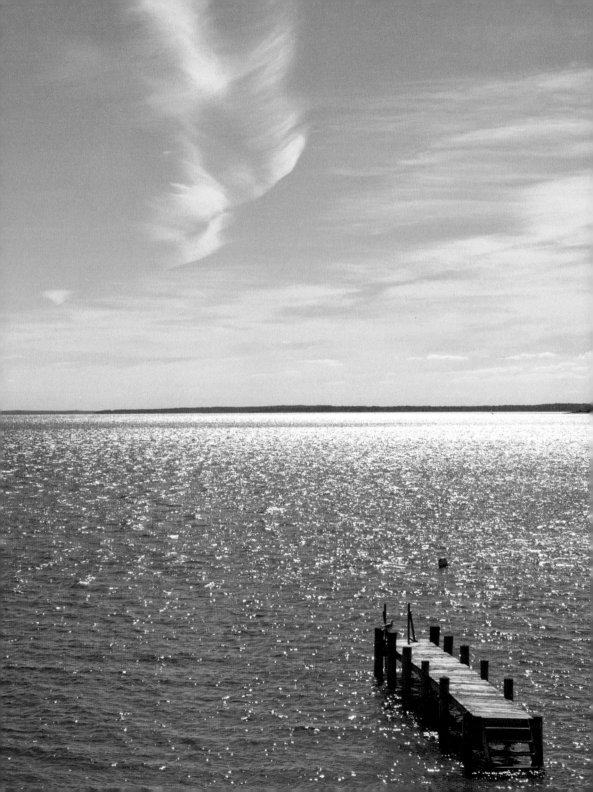

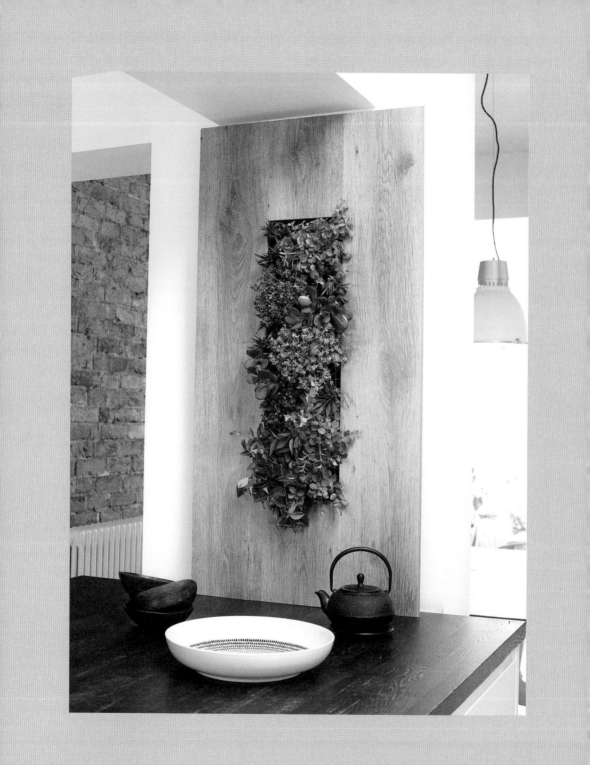

명성 myung sung living meditation

Unlike the previous two meditation tools that are an event unto themselves, Myung Sung proposes the idea of "living meditation," during the act of daily living. This concept was recently introduced in 2022 by Dr. Jenelle Kim in her book *Myung Sung: The Korean Art of Living Meditation*, which explores how meditation can be a continuous overlay on our lives, instead of just another checkbox on our ever-growing to-do lists.

According to Dr. Kim, Myung Sung entails the mastery of eight keys, which include:

1 Knowing and being grounded in our true selves, and delineating who we really are from outside influences.

2 Connecting to our inner self and the best interest of others to balance what is right and true.

3 Widening our perspectives and expanding our thoughts and beliefs to avoid being selfishly "drunk on your own thoughts."

4 Leaving a legacy of goodness over chasing fleeting and materialistic sources of happiness.

5 Living with honor by respecting the multidimensional value of living beings.

6 Becoming grounded in our inner worlds to shape our outer realities instead of being tossed around by the turbulence of uncontrollable external circumstances.

7 Seeking opportunities to garner wisdom from outside circumstances.

8 Going with the flow of natural order and working in harmony with it.

혼족 honjok

Honjok denotes a person who willingly undertakes typical group or couples-oriented activities alone, such as dining and traveling. Popularized within the past decade, Honjok has stimulated a cultural shift that normalizes the act of enjoying activities solo.

Honjok is less intended to categorize or box people into a personality type, but rather to embrace the idea that it's normal to enjoy time alone, and that being alone or single isn't lonely or pitiful. It also relieves individuals from the stress and social expectation of having to get married, or maintain needless and superficial relationships in the midst of an already high-demand life.

Spin-offs of the term Honjok include the following slang terms:

혼밥 **Honbap**
A person who enjoys eating alone

혼술 **Honsul**
A person who enjoys drinking alone

혼놀 **Honnol**
A person who plays, spends time, or conducts leisure activities alone

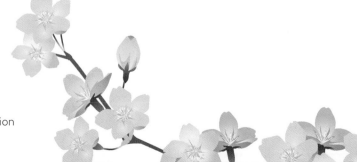

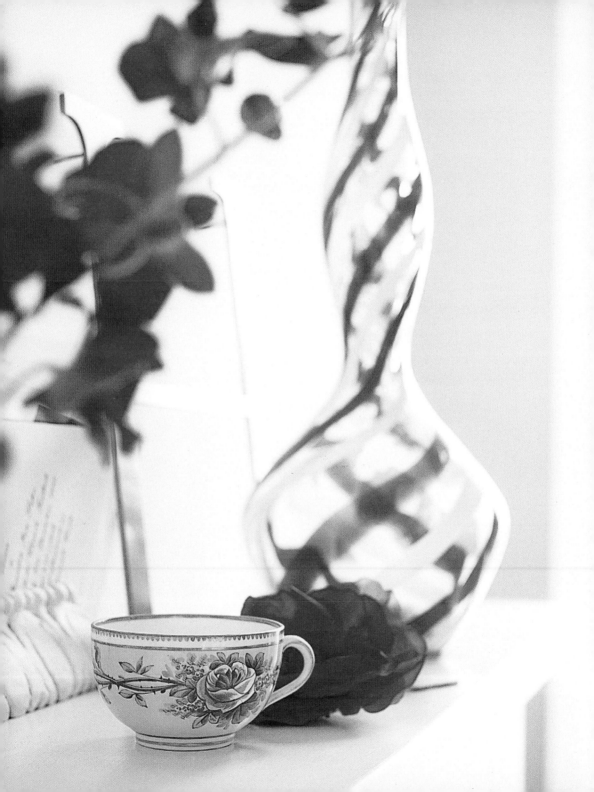

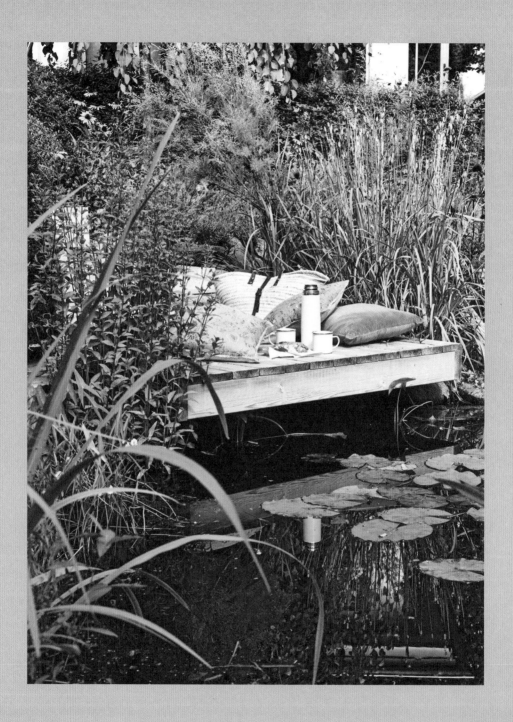

To some, Honjok is interpreted with more depth, as a way of life that achieves a deeper level of self-understanding in spite of some initial solitary discomfort. If this concept appeals to you, here's how to incorporate Honjok into your own life:

1 Normalize the act of doing things by yourself

Abandon the perceived awkwardness of being alone in public. Accept that most people are too busy living their own lives to judge you for being by yourself. Feel liberated in knowing that you can still do everything you feel like doing by yourself. You don't have to wait for anyone to experience life on your own terms. For example, if you want to take yourself out on a date, or celebrate a holiday by yourself, that's okay.

2 Use alone time as a means to reflect

If you find yourself alone against your own wishes, use it as valuable time to look within and develop a deeper understanding of yourself. Once you push past the discomfort of loneliness, you may find that your true thoughts and feelings come to the surface and help you pave a path towards beautifying your inner world.

3 Let go of the pressure to fit society's expectations

Society has built expectations of how we should conduct our time—get married, have a family, balance a social life, and exhibit a healthy dose of extroversion. Although these may be great goalposts for many, it's okay to want to do things on your own terms. Honor your unique self and if that means spending most of your time alone, then so be it.

conclusion

I hope this book has taught you some new self-care tools and tips to add to your arsenal. Whether it's a new skincare hack, a soup recipe, or a mindfulness practice, Korean culture has so much to offer and I've been honored to share these ideas with you.

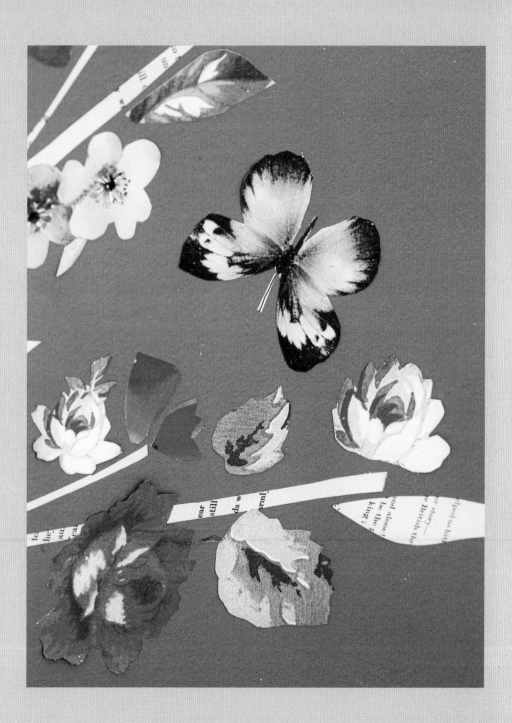

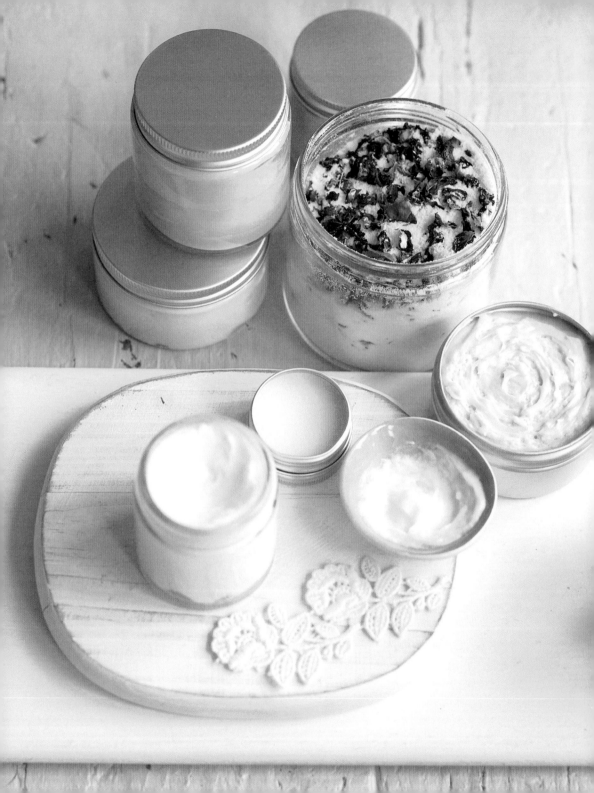

resources

seshin exfoliating mitt

(see page 24)

A simple internet search for "Korean exfoliating mitt" will give you plenty of options for where to purchase these online. Alternatively, a Korean grocer should also carry them. They are manufactured by a variety of brands. Seshin mitts are usually a square-shaped green glove with a few thin black stripes, but they can come in a variety of colors. The cost for a pack of ten ranges from $5–10 US dollars (under £10), although there are higher-end varieties available at a higher price.

skincare products

(see pages 28–32)

As I mentioned in chapter 1, everyone's skin is unique. What works for one person may not work for another. I recommend consulting with an aesthetician or dermatologist to find the best product recommendations suited for your skin type and budget. Experimenting with different products is also an option.

If you don't know where to start, some popular Korean brands are Innisfree, Sulwhasoo, and Laneige. But remember, you don't have to use Korean products to practice the concept of "K-Beauty".

If "clean beauty" (products that tend to have natural, non-synthetic ingredients) is your thing, you can check out Environmental Working Group's Skin Deep Database to search products based on an ingredient assessment: www.ewg.com/skindeep

Here are some products that I'm loving right now. Just a reminder, these are products that work for me personally, and they are not general recommendations. My current focuses are antiaging and clean beauty. I am not a skincare expert. I'm not affiliated with any of these brands, I'm not perfect, and yes I'm still on my own journey of finding what works best for me!

• **Cleanser, serum, and eye cream:** Juice Beauty's Stem Cellular line

• **Other serums:** M-61 Vitablast C Serum 2.0 and Powerglow Pro+ Serum

• **Face oil:** Tata Harper Retinoic Nutrient Face Oil

- **Sunscreen:** Skinceuticals Physical Fusion SPF 50 tinted Sunscreen

- **Night cream:** Jason Vitamin E Age Renewal Moisturizing Cream

- **Mask:** Aztec Secret Indian Healing Clay paired with organic apple cider vinegar (cider vinegar)

Korean food ingredients

(see chapter 2)

Before I share where you can look for each ingredient on this resource list, here are some places to start:

Online:
U.S.:
- www.hmart.com
- www.sayweee.com
- www.sfmart.com
- www.hanyangmart.com

UK and worldwide:
- www.amazon.com
- http://global.gmarket.co.kr/

You can also search for brick-and-mortar Korean grocery stores in your area. These will vary greatly depending on your location.

Asian chives

You will mostly likely not find Asian chives, or buchu (부추) in a regular grocery store. Check out a Korean or Asian grocery store for these.

Fermented Korean sauces

Gochujang, doenjang, and ganjang may all be found in Korean or Asian grocery stores, or in one of the links mentioned on page 134.

With its growing popularity, many conventional grocery stores are also stocking gochujang in their sauce section. Chung Jung and Mother-in-Law are two brands I recommend.

Glutinous rice

Glutinous rice, or chapssal (찹쌀) may be found in Asian groceries, the international section of regular grocery stores, or online. A simple internet query of "sweet glutinous rice" will give you various options.

Gochugaru

These Korean red chili flakes are available in any Korean grocery store and most Asian groceries. Gochugaru can be found in powder form for recipes that require a smooth texture, such as pastes. Many dishes generally call for the flakes, so you'll need to pay close attention to the recipe.

Some brands that produce gochugaru include Taekyung, Mother-in-law, and a variety of others. Keep in mind that the labeling may be written in Korean in Asian grocers, so ask an associate to help you if you don't know Korean.

Korean teas

If you prefer to consume the teas mentioned on pages 84–88 ready-made, some popular Korean tea bag brands are Damtuh, Dongsuh, and Surasang.

Some additional notes:

• **Nogcha (Green tea):** One of Korea's premiere green tea brands is Osulloc. However, there's no need to get fancy—any green tea bag will do.

If you don't have access to a brick-and-mortar Korean grocery, search the following ingredients in any of the links on page 134 for Korean ingredients.

• **Job's tears:** Job's tears may also be referred to as adlay and resembles puffed wheat. It typically comes in a bag or jar.

• **Buckwheat grains**

• **Roasted pearl barley grains**

• **Korean plum extract**

• **Honey citron tea**

• **Dried jujubes**

Miyeok

Miyeok can be found at Korean or Asian groceries. It is typically sold in long bags and appears long and stringy with a deep green hue that looks almost black or charcoal. Alternatively, you may run a search for miyeok or "dried Korean seaweed" and order it online. Note that Miyeok may also be sold under the Japanese name, "wakame." Popular Korean brands for Miyeok are Nonghyup and Chung Jung, although others can be equally as good.

Napa cabbage

Napa cabbage should be available in most supermarkets and grocery stores in all seasons.

Namul (edible grass) growing

Searching for the terms "Korean Natural Farming" or JADAM will connect you with resources on how to grow your own namul at home.

https://en.jadam.kr/
https://christrump.com/

Additional Korean recipes and food blogs

Cookbooks:
- *The Kimchi Cookbook* by Lauryn Chun
- *Koreatown: A Cookbook* by Deuki Hong and Matt Rodbard
- *Maangchi's Big Book of Korean Cooking* by Maangchi
- *The Korean Vegan Cookbook* by Joanne Lee Molinaro
- *Korean Mother's Easy Recipes* by Yoon Okhee
- *Wookwan's Korean Temple Food* by Wookwan

Korean food blogs:
- www.maanchi.com
- www.mykoreankitchen.com
- www.koreanbapsang.com
- www.kimchimari.com

Forest bathing
Book:
- *Forest Bathing* by Dr. Qing Li

Meditation
For more information on the meditation practices on pages 118–125, see:

Maum Su-ryun Meditation:
www.woomyung.com

Kuok Sundo Breathing:
www.sundointernational.com

Myung Sung Living Meditation:
Myung Sung (book) by Dr. Jenelle Kim

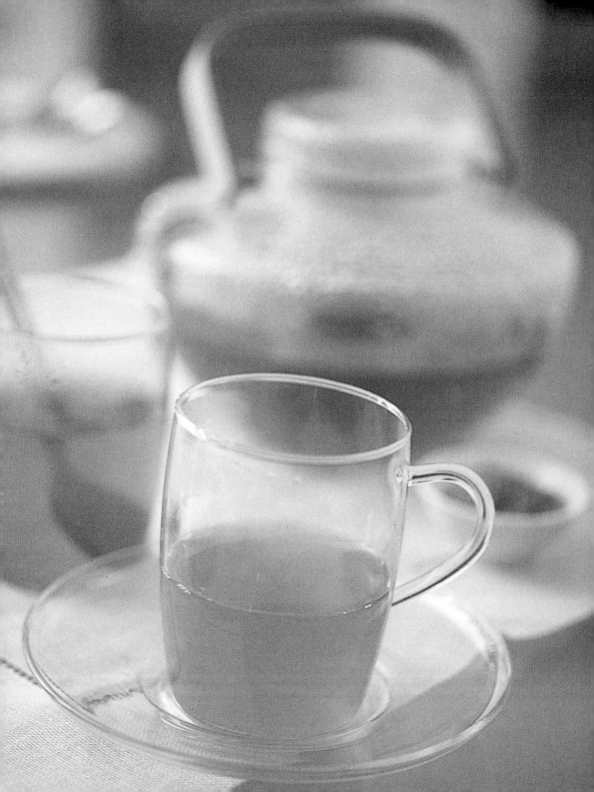

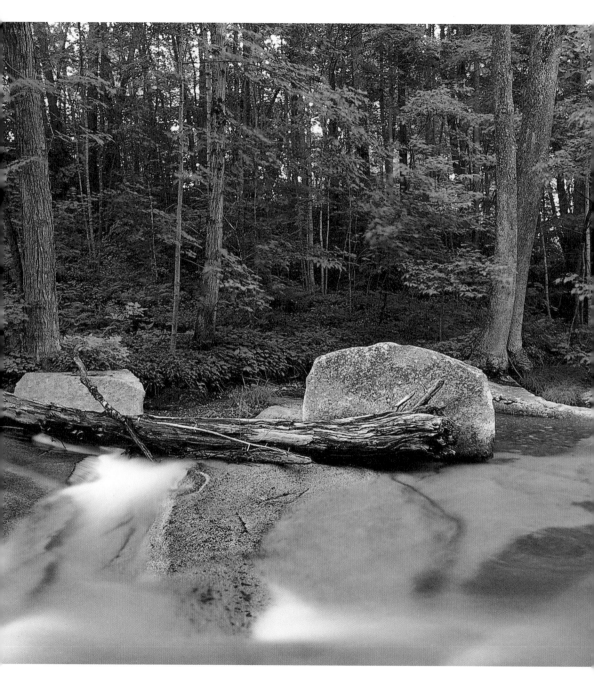

index

Picture credits

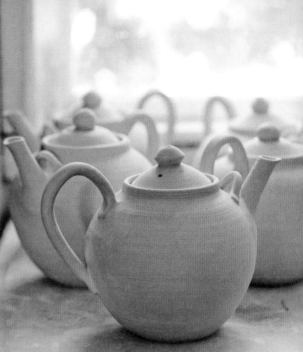

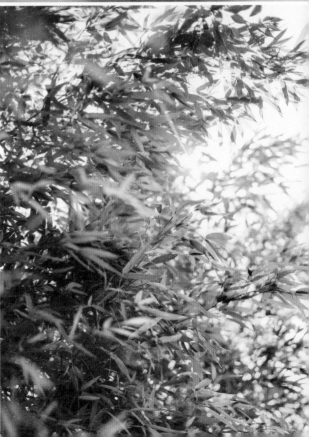

about Isa

Isa Kujawski is a functional dietitian nutritionist, wellness expert, and U.S. Navy veteran. As a biracial half-Korean, she grew up in the melting pot of New York City where her immigrant parents met while taking English classes. Her ancestry traces back to the northern parts of Korea where her grandparents fled communism in war-torn Korea to ensure a better life for their descendants.

Growing up exclusively around the Korean side of her family, Isa was raised speaking Korean as her first language, eating Korean food as her staple cuisine, and hearing her mother's stories about how her late grandmother made legendary homemade kimchi for her ten children.

In 2011, she had the opportunity to be stationed in Seoul, South Korea as a U.S. Naval Officer for two years and experience first-hand the richness of Korean culture and the depth of Korea's unique self-care practices, which she is proud to have the opportunity to share with the world.

Isa currently runs her own company Mea Nutrition, which focuses on food as medicine, nutritional psychology, and holistic healing. Her mission is to help chronically stressed individuals, especially her fellow veterans, rebalance their mind and body through the healing power of nutrition. Connecting nutrition with mental wellbeing, Isa aims to help people feel alive again and find true wealth through vibrant health. As a sought-after source, she has been featured in Mind Body Green, Shape, Food & Nutrition, VeryWell, Thrive, Eat This, and Livestrong. You can find Isa at www.meanutrition.com.

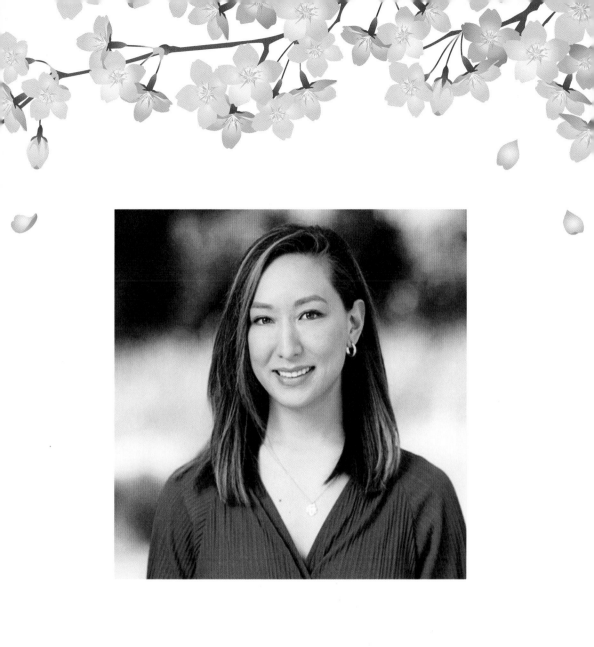

acknowledgments

Thank you to my family, who courageously took multiple leaps of faith in the face of trials and tribulations. It's because of you that I had the opportunity to grow up multiculturally, and that's a gift. Without you I would not have been qualified to write this book.

Thank you to my dear friend Seongyoon Cho, who graciously showed me around Korea, helped me expand my Korean vocabulary, and helped me laugh when life got tough. Your contributions to both this book and my time in Korea will never be forgotten.

To my friend Gian—thank you for always inspiring me with your grit, tenacity, and creative mind. You are a version of myself I want to become someday, and being like you is a goal worth aspiring to.

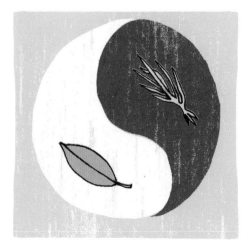